The Arrhythmic Patient in the Emergency Department

Massimo Zecchin • Gianfranco Sinagra
Editors

The Arrhythmic Patient in the Emergency Department

A Practical Guide for Cardiologists and Emergency Physicians

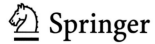 Springer

Editors
Massimo Zecchin
Cardiovascular Department
Cattinara University Hospital
Trieste
Italy

Gianfranco Sinagra
Cardiovascular Department
Cattinara University Hospital
Trieste
Italy

ISBN 978-3-319-24326-9   ISBN 978-3-319-24328-3   (eBook)
DOI 10.1007/978-3-319-24328-3

Library of Congress Control Number: 2015958251

Springer Cham Heidelberg New York Dordrecht London

Printed on acid-free paper

Springer International Publishing AG Switzerland is part of Springer Science+Business Media
(www.springer.com)

Foreword

Treatment of patients with cardiovascular diseases has dramatically changed over the past 20 years. Accompanied by an incredible increase in pathophysiological understanding and availability of treatment options, specialized fields of expertise have rapidly evolved.

Electrophysiology is one of these newcomers. Based on the analysis of basic principles of electrical activation in the human heart, the field has developed into sophisticated treatment strategies of device therapy and catheter ablation. The majorities of today's EP patients originate from the mainstream of everyday clinical cardiology and present with endemic, bradycardic, and tachycardic arrhythmias.

With this background, electrophysiology has also arrived in the ER department.

Now it is our obligation to transport our knowledge and expertise for treatment of arrhythmia patients to our cardiology colleagues and specialized ER physicians who encounter emergency situations due to or accompanied by cardiac arrhythmias in a significant number of patients, next to a variety of other medical emergencies.

Dedicated literature on that topic is really scarce. I therefore want to thank the editors and authors of this book to take the challenge, efforts, and work and to bring together a vast amount of EP knowledge and to focus it to the special situation in the ER.

This book should become an integral part of training for young cardiology fellows, and it will be a practical guide and help for all medical staff involved into the management of ER patients.

Christopher Piorkowski
Head of EP Department – University of Dresden

Preface

The book is a practical guide designed for physicians (both emergency physicians and cardiologists) who first evaluate and treat patients with arrhythmias or potentially arrhythmic problems in the emergency setting. It can also be a useful learning tool for students and residents in Cardiology and Emergency Medicine.

In all chapters, every effort was made to provide a brief but comprehensive summary of the topic with both theoretical and practical suggestions, considering the different needs of the specialists involved in the primary care of arrhythmic patients.

The diagnostic pathways and treatment options of patients presenting in the Emergency Department with syncope or arrhythmias, including bradyarrhythmias, atrial fibrillation, and narrow and wide QRS tachycardias, are discussed. In addition, clear advice for the management of patients with cardiac devices and possible dysfunction, electrical storm, or a requirement for urgent surgery are provided.

Practical suggestions are offered for short-term management, e.g., regarding the decision on when to hospitalize the patient and some hints for long-term pharmacological and non-pharmacological treatment.

In the first chapter, an overview of the management of arrhythmic patients, from the emergency physician's point of view, is provided. In the second chapter, some considerations, beyond published guidelines, for the management of syncope are given by a leading expert. An extensive theoretical overview of brady- and tachyarrhythmias are then followed by practical flowcharts in Chaps. 3, 4 and 5, while in the following chapter the differential diagnosis of wide-QRS tachycardias with clear examples are discussed by one of the greatest experts in this field. Chapters 7 and 8 deal with quite rare cardiac conditions, sometimes not so known by emergency physicians and even by cardiologists, who nonetheless in such cases sometimes face difficult decisions. Differently, situations frequently observed in the Emergency Department, but with an arrhythmogenic potential which is not always well defined, are presented in Chaps. 9 and 10. Finally, in the last three chapters, some indications for the management of patients with implanted cardiac devices presenting in Emergency Department or who need urgent surgery are provided, again considering the different skills of the various medical figures involved in the primary care of such patients.

Considering the heterogeneity of the topics, some differences in the chapters' frameworks were necessary. However, the book was conceived to offer quick information and solutions to the single issues, as required in the emergency setting, rather than providing a systematic review.

Trieste, Italy   Massimo Zecchin
                                                                                                       Gianfranco Sinagra

Contents

Management of Arrhythmic Patients in the Emergency Department: General Principles

1

Alessandro Surian and Luca Visintin

Arrhythmic patients are common in the duty of the emergency physician and the cardiology consultant. Both specialists, with their different approach and method, well know the clinical and statistical relevance of arrhythmias.

A wide range of symptoms leading the patient to the emergency department may be related to a cardiac rhythm disorder. They may vary from simple palpitations to a cardiac arrest. Otherwise, the diagnosis of arrhythmia can be made in patients who came to the ED for other diseases.

Emergency physician is the first doctor approaching the patient and must initially define the hemodynamic state induced by the arrhythmia. The need to assure hemodynamic stability must be assumed as the first important target and should not be delayed by any other consideration.

Once a stabilization is obtained, the consultant cardiologist can improve diagnostic and therapeutic definition. A tight cooperation between the two specialists warrants the best patient outcome.

1.1 Triage

Triage of arrhythmic patient must focus on hemodynamic state and time of onset of symptoms and signs. Unstable arrhythmias should be admitted as soon as possible to physician evaluation, while asymptomatic patients may wait longer.

A. Surian (✉) • L. Visintin
Emergency Medicine Unit, Cardiovascular Department,
Cattinara University Hospital, Trieste, Italy
e-mail: dottalesurian@yahoo.it

© Springer International Publishing Switzerland 2016
M. Zecchin, G. Sinagra (eds.), *The Arrhythmic Patient in the Emergency
Department: A Practical Guide for Cardiologists and Emergency Physicians*,
DOI 10.1007/978-3-319-24328-3_1

Hemodynamic criteria for quick admission are:

- SBP (systolic blood pressure): <90 mmHg
- DBP (diastolic blood pressure): <60 mmHg
- Heart rate per minute: >120 and <50 bpm
- Respiratory rate per minute: >30 and <10
- Body temperature: >39.0 °C and <36.0 °C
- Sat O_2: <90 %

Moreover, chest pain, dyspnea, acute heart failure, acute altered mental status, and signs of shock are evaluated during triage.

Unstable patients should be addressed immediately to the shock room of the ED, while stable patient can wait or be addressed to an examination room provided with ECG for a first evaluation and subsequently be treated when the adequate setting is available [1, 2].

1.2 Emergency Department Physician Approach to the Arrhythmic Patient

Emergency physician's main task is to identify "*hemodynamically unstable*" patients, quickly evaluating parameters like level of consciousness, ventilation, oxygenation, heart rate, and blood pressure (Table 1.1). Clinical evaluation is focused on the investigation of signs of shock (altered mental status, cool and clammy skin, weak and rapid pulse, rapid and shallow breathing, anxiety, lightheadedness, chest pain, decrease of urine, thirst and dry mouth, hypoglycemia, confusion, nausea, lackluster eyes) dyspnea and tachypnea, or oxygen desaturation.

Patient's ECG, blood pressure, and O_2 saturation (sat O_2) should be immediately put under continuous monitoring and intravenous line with blood samples provided. Airways have to be kept patent, breathing assisted, and oxygen given if sat O_2 is below 94 %. A 12-lead ECG should be obtained as soon as possible for a correct diagnostic evaluation of the arrhythmia. Medical history must be gathered.

Table 1.1 First steps	
Look for:
shock signs
Chest pain
Respiratory distress
Do:
Monitor the patient, IV line, blood samples
Ensure patent airway and ventilation and give oxygen (if needed)
Support perfusion pressure (use mean arterial pressure as a good index)
12-leads ECG; gather medical history
Treat reversible causes

Should a cardiac arrest occure, advanced life support protocols have to be applied.

Hemodynamic instability, defined as an acute organ failure or a near-cardiac arrest situation, may be due to tachy- or bradyarrhythmia.

In the event of a tachyarrhythmia, an immediate defibrillation or synchronized cardioversion should be done regardless of the arrhythmia mechanism.

In addition, bradyarrhythmias may lead to a severe decrease in cardiac output, causing hemodynamic instability with hypotension, mental dizziness, decreased consciousness level, cyanosis, dyspnea, etc.

A treatment based on atropine, catecholamine, or an electrical stimulation may be helpful or even lifesaver [1, 2].

1.2.1 Tachyarrhythmia

By definition, tachycardia is a heart rate exceeding 100 beats per minute.

By far the most common tachycardia diagnosed in the emergency department is sinus tachycardia.

In the healthy patient, it is a physiological response to physical stress or anxiety. Sinus tachycardia is also a normal condition during the pregnancy. In most other cases, it is due to an underlying pathological condition (e.g., fever, dehydration, anemia and hypoxia, ACS, P.E., hyperthyroidism, high blood pressure, smoking, alcohol, beverages containing caffeine, medication side effects, abuse of recreational drugs, such as cocaine, or imbalance of electrolytes) [3].

"Appropriate" sinus tachycardia offsets an underlying condition, while "inappropriate" sinus tachycardia can be a consequence of deficit of vagal tonus or a hyperactivity of/excessive sensibility to the sympathetic nervous system. During sinus tachycardia heart rate is usually lower than 140–150 bpm, even if, in young people under extreme stimulation, it can exceed 220 bpm. Typically, in sinus tachycardia, the P wave is positive in inferior and lateral leads (as in sinus rhythm). As sympathetic activation increases AV conduction, PR interval is shorter than in sinus rhythm; therefore, with few exceptions, the coexistence of long PR and sinus tachycardia is unlikely, even in patients with I degree AV block during normal sinus rhythm, and usually suggests other mechanisms of tachycardia, as atrial tachycardia or atrial flutter, possibly with 2:1 conduction and a P wave hidden within the QRS complex.

In order to identify if the tachycardia is the main cause of the patient's symptoms, a complete physical examination, blood draw to test metabolic and renal function, emogasanalysis (EGA), 12-lead ECG results and medical history should be performed and any potential reversible causes should be corrected.

Usually tachycardia may be considered as hemodynamically significant when they exceed 150 bpm.

However, it is important to remark that even frequencies lower than 150 bpm may cause hemodynamic compromise, mainly if it is sustained for a prolonged time and/or coexists with an underlying heart disease, leading to chest pain, altered mental status, pulmonary edema, or cardiogenic shock, requiring an emergency electrical cardioversion.

It is advised to perform an effective pre-procedural sedation if the patient is conscious, although hemodynamically unstable.

1.2.1.1 Procedural Sedation/Anesthesia During Cardioversion

Sedative or dissociative drugs, coupled with or analgesics, are used to relieve the patient from unpleasant procedures. Many of these drugs can lead to central nervous system and cardiac and/or respiratory depression. Given the potential risks, regulatory agencies are debating about the medical privileges needed to perform this procedure, particularly about the presence of an anesthesiologist during the procedure.

Recommendations for a safe employ consist of a proper setting (ECG, respiratory rate, sat O2, NIBP monitoring, advance life support trained personnel, devices for life support) and frequent reevaluations (prior to, during, and after procedure); trained staff should choose appropriate drugs and dosing depending on the distinctive features of each patient.

A growing literature highlights the safety of administration of ketamine, midazolam, fentanyl, propofol, and etomidate in the ED [4–6].

- *Equipment and supplies*: oxygen, suction, reversal agents, advanced life support medications and equipment, defibrillator, and CO_2 capnography. An IV line should be set; reversal agents should be available whenever opioids and benzodiazepines are administered.
- *Personnel*: during the procedure, personnel dedicated to patient monitoring should focus only to the sedation and not to other tasks.
- *Training*: the physician should know drug's pharmacology of the agents used and their antagonists. Personnel with experience in Advanced Cardiac Life Support should be present.
- *Drugs*. Electrical cardioversion is a brief but painful procedure. Light sedation is inadequate for a pain-free relaxed patient. Therefore, a moderate to deep sedation and analgesia or general anesthesia is required. In most US and Europe hospitals, emergency physicians are not allowed to provide general anesthesia, so sedation can be the only option if an anesthesiologist is not present. Drugs: midazolam and fentanyl are commonly used, but their long-lasting effects make them not handy or straight dangerous. Instead, for a brief and titratable deep sedation, it makes more sense to employ propofol, etomidate, or methohexital combined with fentanyl. There are contradictory statements from the American Society of Anesthesiologists (ASA) guidelines about authorization for propofol use by emergency physicians. Evidence is accumulating that non-anesthesiologist-administered propofol sedation has a safety and efficacy profile comparable or superior to that provided by benzodiazepines with or without opioids. Medications should be administered gradually, allowing sufficient time between dose and effect assessment. Concurrent administration of sedative and analgesic drugs requires evaluation on dose reduction.
- *Recovery*: observation should be prolonged until there are no more risks for cardiorespiratory depression. Medical institution should set up appropriate discharge criteria [4–6].

1.2.1.2 Cardioversion/Defibrillation

If cardioversion is chosen, set the defibrillator into the synchronized mode. This to avoid shock delivery during ventricular "electric vulnerability" period (apex and descending branch of T wave), a potential trigger of ventricular fibrillation. Defibrillation, used for interruption of pulseless VT, VF, and torsade de pointes synchronization, should be avoided, as QRS complexes may not be identified.

Emergency physician should be trained to recognize the presence of the P wave and distinguish between narrow-complex (supraventricular) tachycardia and wide complex tachycardia, which in condition of urgency should be considered and treated as ventricular tachycardia.

The different types of tachycardia can be treated with different energies:

- As recommended by international guidelines for regular narrow-complex tachycardia, the initial energy cardioversion should be 50–100 J with biphasic defibrillators and 200 J if monophasic (Class IIa, LOE B).
- For irregular narrow-complex tachycardia, the recommended initial biphasic energy is 120–200 J (Class IIa; LOE A).
- Regular wide complex tachycardia may resolve after discharge at 100 J by both biphasic and monophasic defibrillators (Class IIb, LOE C).

Anyway, if the first shock is inadequate to resolve the arrhythmia, increase energy "in a stepwise fashion."

When using monophasic defibrillators, initial energy should be set to 200 J, proceeding in a stepwise fashion in the event of failure.

The irregular wide complex tachycardia should be treated with high-energy unsynchronized shock (i.e., defibrillation), because of the difficulty of the machine to distinguish between the QRS complex and T wave.

Even if there were doubts whether the tachycardia is monomorphic or polymorphic, the shock should not be delayed and a high-energy unsynchronized shock must be delivered.

In the unstable patient (if not hypotensive) presenting with a regular narrow QRS complex tachycardia, *adenosine* is safe to be used while cardiac electrical cardioversion is being set up both for therapeutic (in case of tachycardia involving the AV node as a part of the reentry circuit) and diagnostic (in case of atrial arrhythmias, unmasking atrial activity slowing AV conduction (Class IIb (LOE C)).

If the patient with tachycardia is stable, the emergency physician will have more time for a correct diagnosis and to choose the most appropriate therapy, with the help of a cardiologist if necessary.

After obtaining a complete medical history and a careful physical examination, QRS complex evaluation is needed. QRS duration should be measured in at least two orthogonal derivations: narrow-complex tachycardia (QRS duration <120 ms) should be always considered, by definition, as supraventricular: examples are sinus tachycardia, atrial fibrillation (AF), atrial flutter, AV nodal reentrant tachyarrhythmia (AVNRT), tachyarrhythmia mediated by accessory pathways, atrial tachycardia, multifocal atrial tachycardia (MAT), and junctional tachycardia (rare in adults) .

Based on ECG findings, the regularity of RR intervals and the relationship between P waves and QRS complexes along with the timing of onset of tachycardia may help to differentiate among the various kinds of supraventricular tachyarrhythmia.

If the anamnesis highlights sudden onset of palpitations and its rapid resolution, it is likely to be atrial fibrillation, atrial flutter, AVNRT, atrioventricular reciprocating tachycardia, and atrial tachycardia. Instead, sinus tachycardia, permanent atrial fibrillation, and permanent flutter, together with MAT and premature atrial contractions, show symptoms that arise and resolved more gradually [7].

P waves immediately preceding the QRS complexes address the ED physician's diagnosis to sinus tachycardia, atrial tachycardia, multifocal atrial tachycardia or multiple atrial premature contractions.

P waves following QRS complexes suggest atrioventricular nodal reentrant tachycardia, atrioventricular reciprocating tachycardia, or atrial tachycardia. However, heart rate can be high enough to have T waves overlapping the P waves.

If tachycardia has a narrow QRS complex, vagal maneuvers and, if ineffective, the administration of adenosine at doses of 6–12 mg, (always under cardiac monitoring) may have a dual purpose:

- *Diagnostic*, since the increase of degree of AV block can unmask the nature of the underlying rhythm; a transient slowing of ventricular rate may highlight atrial fibrillation, atrial flutter, and sinus tachycardia, while there might not be any effect on multifocal atrial tachycardia or frequent atrial premature contractions.
- *Therapeutic*, because the increase in parasympathetic tone may slow electrical conduction through the AV node interrupting reentrant arrhythmias involving tissues sensitive to vagal stimulation (AV nodal reentrant tachycardia, AV reciprocating tachycardia, and sometimes atrial tachycardia).

If vagal maneuvers and adenosine are unsuccessful in converting to sinus rhythm or atrial fibrillation and atrial flutter are diagnosed, it is recommended to administer:

- *Diltiazem* (15–20 mg or 0.25 mg/kg IV over 2 min); if needed, after 15 min an additional IV dose of 20–25 mg (0.35 mg/kg) can be administered; the infusion dose is 5–15 mg/h, titrated according to heart rate.
- *Verapamil* (2.5–5 mg IV bolus over 2 min); if no response and non-drug-induced adverse events occur, it is possible to repeat doses of 5–10 mg every 15–30 min up to a total dose of 20 mg.
- *Beta-blockers* (metoprolol, atenolol, propranolol, esmolol, and labetalol).

These drugs are able to convert the reentrant tachycardia by acting on the nodal tissue or slowing the ventricular response in case of other supraventricular arrhythmias [1].

In patients with atrial fibrillation/flutter/tachycardia lasting more than 48 h (or if the onset of the arrhythmia is unknown), electrical or pharmacological cardioversion should not be attempted in absence of adequate anticoagulation in the preceding 3 weeks. Otherwise, when prompt restoring of sinus rhythm is needed or preferred, cardioversion can be done after excluding the presence of thrombi in the left atrium by transesophageal echocardiography (Class IIa, LOE B) [8].

In most cases the patient with narrow QRS tachycardia is treated in ED, restoring the RS or starting a therapy aimed to control the heart rate, and resigned to be entrusted to the outpatient cardiologist, who will complete the diagnostic process and improve, if necessary, the treatment started in the emergency department.

Handling of wide-QRS complex tachycardia (>120 ms) is different. These tachy-cardias cannot be treated in PS only but require both an initial cardiac evaluation in the emergency department, including a careful analysis of the ECG and echocar-diography, and hospitalization in the specialist department.

1.2.1.3 When should the Cardiology Consultant be called?

Cardiologist called in ED for a patient with a wide-QRS complex tachycardia has a daunting task. In fact, a mistaken diagnostic may lead to disastrous effects in terms of prognosis.

A wide-complex tachycardia can be:

- Ventricular tachycardia.
- Supraventricular tachycardia in a patient with preexisting bundle branch block.
- Tachycardia-dependent bundle branch block (aberrancy).
- Tachycardia caused by drug that have a widening effect on QRS.
- Atrial arrhythmias in the presence of ventricular pre-excitation.

In the diagnostic path of a wide-QRS complex tachycardia, attention must be paid to the clinical examination (variability of the first tone and amplitude variable radial pulse lay for the presence of AV dissociation) and the careful analysis of the ECG [9].

Here is a summary of some general criteria that can help the cardiologist identify the origin of tachycardia (for detailed discussion of the ECG, see Chap. 6):

A. Search if the electrical activity of the atria is present; P waves, independent of QRS, are separated by constant intervals, paying more attention in derivation II and V1, where these waves can be easier to find.

 If some ventricular impulses are not conducted to the atria and the QRS/P ratio is greater than 1, a diagnosis of ventricular tachycardia can be made.

 Small deflections, fitting in a rhythmic manner inside the QRS complexes, suggest the presence of underlying sinus P waves when their rate is lower than the ventricular rate. Hence, a diagnosis of ventriculoatrial dissociation and therefore of ventricular tachycardia can be made. If there is a mathematical rela-tionship between ventricular and atrial electrical activity, a retrograde ventricular-atrial conduction is likely, as it can be found in about 50 % of cases..

 In presence of a clear QRS/P ratio = 1, the diagnosis may be more difficult; it may be expression of atrial tachycardia, sinus rhythm with aberrant conduction, nodal reentrant tachycardia, automatic junctional tachycardia, reciprocating orthodromic tachycardia with aberrant conduction, or ventricular tachycardia with 1:1 retrograde conduction.

B. Search for "concordance" aspect of QRS in the precordial leads. The presence of concordance suggests that the tachycardia has a ventricular origin. Common definitions are "*positive concordance*" if the QRS complex is "R wavelike" from V1 to V6 and "*negative concordance*" in the presence of a "QS-like" morphology from V1 to V6.

Cardiologists must remember that although a negative concordance is absolutely specific for VT, the positive could, in rare cases, be expression of a pre-excited tachycardia due to a left posterior Kent bundle (pre-excited tachycardia with conduction through ancillary pathway).

C. As stated by Brugada et al., in the diagnostic algorithm of regular wide-QRS complex tachycardia, the presence of RS complexes (R waves followed by S wave) in precordial leads suggests a diagnosis of VT when the interval between the beginning of the R wave and nadir of the S wave is >100 ms [10].

D. The analysis of QRS complexes, in particular in leads V1 and V6, is certainly useful.

In a wide-QRS complex tachycardia with right bundle branch block (positive QRS in V1), morphologies R, Rs, RrÐ, qR in V1 and QS, qR, rS in V6 are suggestive of ventricular tachycardia.

A three-phasic morphology of V1 (rsR' and rSR'), biphasic morphology in V1 (rRÐ), or three-phasic morphologies in V6 (qRs) suggest a supraventricular genesis with aberrant conduction.

In wide-QRS complex tachycardia with left bundle branch block (negative QRS in V1), an initial R wave >30 ms in V1, an interval between the beginning of the QRs complex and nadir of the S wave >60 ms, the presence of a notch in the descending limb of the S wave, and Q wave in V6 (qR aspects, QRS or QS) suggest a ventricular origin of arrhythmia.

Initial R wave <30 ms and an interval between the QRS onset and the S wave nadir <60 ms are suggestive of supraventricular tachycardia with aberrant conduction.

The maneuvers of vagal stimulation can be useful in the diagnosis of wide complex tachycardia, and depending on the response, we can obtain important information:

- If the tachycardia ceases, a supraventricular reentrant tachycardia is likely (but in some cases even the idiopathic ventricular tachycardia is resolved with the vagal stimulation).
- Modifications of the atrioventricular conduction in atrial tachycardia and atrial flutter can be observed.
- In ventricular tachycardia with ventriculoatrial (VA) 1:1 conduction, a variation of VA interval or transient second-degree retrograde VA block may be recorded.

1.2.1.4 Treatment of a Wide-QRS Complex Tachycardia

As mentioned earlier, if the patient gets worse and becomes unstable, staff must be ready to perform an *immediate electrical cardioversion* or to deliver high-energy unsynchronized shock, if ventricular fibrillation emerges or instability is caused by a polymorphic VT.

When diagnostic doubts about the origin of tachycardia are present, it should be treated as if it were of ventricular origin.

In presence of regular and monomorphic complexes, it is reasonable to administer *adenosine*, considered safe, and useful for both diagnosis and treatment purposes (Class IIb, LOE B). Adenosine should not be administered if the patient is unstable or has irregular or polymorphic complexes: in this condition, it could lead to degeneration in VF (Class III, LOE C).

Once diagnosed a ventricular tachycardia, treatment consists of antiarrhythmic drugs such as *procainamide* (Class IIa, LOE B), *amiodarone* (Class IIb, LOE B), or *sotalol* (Class IIb, LOE B) or *electrical cardioversion*.

In patients with known long QT during sinus rhythm, procainamide and sotalol should be avoided.

Procainamide is administered in the initial dose of 10 mg/kg, at rate of 20–50 mg/min. Maximum dose is 17 mg/kg. Maintenance infusion is 1–4 mg/min.

Amiodarone is given 150 mg IV over 10 min; dosing should be repeated to a maximum dose of 2.2 g IV for 24 h.

If an antiarrhythmic drug was already administered without success, it is advisable not to use a second drug without a cardiologist consult (Class III, LOE B) or proceed with electrical cardioversion (Class IIa, LOE C).

Lidocaine is now considered a drug of second choice for the treatment of ventricular tachycardia (dose: 1–1.5 mg/kg IV bolus). Maintenance infusion is 1–4 mg/kg (30–50 mcg/kg per min).

If the wide-QRS complex tachycardia is irregular, the underlying rhythm is likely to be an atrial fibrillation with aberrant conduction. In this case some considerations about the best treatment (rate control or rhythm control) are necessary, in particular:

- Avoid cardioversion if the arrhythmia has been present for more than 48 h (and the patient is stable enough). Consider treatment options with the consultant cardiologist, in particular transesophageal echocardiography to exclude the presence of a thrombus in the left atrium.
- Administer IV *heparin* before cardioversion if not contraindicated.

Irregular polymorphic tachycardia needs an immediate defibrillation. Drugs that may prolong the QT interval should be withdrawn and serum electrolytes corrected.

Myocardial ischemia is the most common cause of polymorphic VT in absence of a prolonged QT interval. In this circumstance amiodarone and sotalol are able to reduce the recurrence of the arrhythmia (Class IIb, LOE C).

1.2.2   Bradycardia

A heart rate below 60 bpm is usually defined as bradycardia. While in young healthy subjects and particularly in athletes it can be a common and non-suspect remark, it can conceal various kinds of diseases.

Usual symptoms of bradycardia are asthenia, fatigue, dyspnea, chest discomfort or pain, pre- or complete loss of consciousness, light-headedness, and decreased level of consciousness. Signs often noticeable are hypotension and/or orthostatic hypotension, diaphoresis, bradycardia-related (escape) frequent premature ventricular complexes, or other ventricular tachyarrhythmias. All the signs and symptoms are due to the discrepancy between the low heart rate and the metabolic requests of the organism.

Usually symptoms are relevant when lower than 40 bpm or higher in presence of a pre- or coexistent cardiac disease [1, 2, 11–13].

First approach: whatever is the underlying cause, ED physician must define the hemodynamic compensation. If low heart rate is the cause of the symptoms, the patient should be immediately treated with drugs and percutaneous or transvenous pacing. The consultant cardiologist should be called to provide support to the diagnosis and treatment.

If the bradycardia is asymptomatic or the hemodynamic condition is acceptable, the thorough diagnosis can be ruled out with more smoothness.

As soon as possible, a 12-lead ECG should be obtained, with a long stripe in II or V1, to unmask atrial activity, for example, the presence of not-detected 2:1 AV block. A complete physical examination and blood tests for troponin, drugs, electrolytes, and serum creatinine must be performed in the meanwhile. If available, an echocardiogram should be used. Chest X-rays or thoracic echography can help to clear up pulmonary edema or congestive heart failure [1, 2, 11, 12].

Based on the ECG findings, we can discern the following rhythms:

1.2.3 Sinus Bradycardia

It can be a sign of underlying pathologies (e.g., vagal hypertonia, drug effect, hypoxia, ischemia of sinoatrial node due to occlusion of right coronary arteria, etc.).

ECG shows a regular sinus rhythm with heart rate lower than 60 bpm and a constant 1:1 AV conduction with PR interval of 120–200 ms (in the absence of coexistent AV block); P waves are regular, with identical waveform, axis between 0 and 90°.

Symptoms can be absent at rest and may appear only during effort.

Common causes are listed in Table 1.2.

Table 1.2 Common causes of sinus bradycardia

Vagal stimulus	Vomit, abdominal pain (i.e., acute retention of urine, acute abdomen, aortic aneurysm), Valsalva maneuver, carotid sinus hypersensitivity
Drugs	β-blockers, Ca^{++} channel blockers, ivabradine, digoxin, amiodarone, quinidine, and virtually all the antiarrhythmic drugs
Hyperkalemia	Acute or chronic heart failure, ACE-I or K+ savers drugs
Hypothermia	
Hypothyroidism	Autoimmune diseases, inappropriate levothyroxine dosage in known hypothyroidism
Endocranial hypertension	Acute endocranial hemorrhage
Sinoatrial node hypoperfusion	Right coronary ischemia
Sinoatrial sick syndrome	

It is clear from the analysis of the abovementioned causes how crucial it is to find the underlying etiology of the sinus bradycardia [14].

1.2.4   Pitfalls

Not maintaining a high and broad index of suspicion for underlying causes

1.2.5   Low-Rate Atrial Fibrillation

It is characterized by the absence of recognizable P wave, irregular RR intervals, and narrow or wide QRS complexes depending on the previous history of the patient.

Most common causes are drugs (as most antiarrhythmic drugs, digoxin, β-blockers, Ca^{++} antagonists), especially in older patients with reduced renal and/ or liver function, vagal hypertonia (mainly in young subjects), or atrioventricular (AV) block. The presence of complete AV block ventricular rate is regular, because of junctional (usually at about 35 bpm) or infrahisian ventricular escape (<30 bpm).

Treatment of symptomatic extreme bradycardia consists in drugs (amines) or transcutaneous or intracardiac transvenous pacing to reach hemodynamic stability.

In elderly patients the most bradyarrhythmias are drug related and will wear off as the involved drugs (e.g., digoxin, β -blocker) wash out; in some cases consider starting with atropine followed by amines [7].

1.2.6   Sinus Node Dysfunction: Sick Sinus Syndrome

Sick sinus syndrome is a condition characterized by a wide spectrum of rhythm disturbances: bradycardia, sinusal arrest, paroxysmal atrial tachycardia, and brady-cardia/asystole.

Clinical appearance ranges from asthenia, mental dizziness to syncope, vertigo, and cardiac failure.

Common causes are idiopathic degeneration of sinoatrial node and/or the atrial conduction tissue, right coronary ischemia, and flogistic and infiltrative diseases. More often drugs can be blamed, as beta-blockers, digoxin, Class I and III antiarrhythmic agents, and Ca++ channel blockers.

Tricyclic antidepressant, 4-phosphodyesterase inhibitors and Beta stimulant may induce atrial tachyarrhythmia.

Diagnosis can be reached by anamnesis, ECG, dynamic ECG (Holter, loop recorder), and electrophysiological study (endocavitary or transesophageal).

Depending on the prevalence of tachy- or bradycardia and the underlying cardiac disease, the therapy can vary from drugs to definitive pacing.

Indications for pacemaker implant are symptoms related to bradycardia.

1.2.7   Atrioventricular (AV) Blocks

AV blocks are commonly caused by:

- Lesions of the electrical conduction system of the heart (necrosis, fibrosis, sclerosis)
- Vagal hypertonia (inferior acute myocardial infarction, hypersensitivity of carotidal sinus, vagal maneuvers, abdominal pain, etc.)
- Increase of the refractory period (drugs)

Based on clinical and ECG findings, AV blocks are divided into:

- First-degree AV block (*prolonged* AV conduction *without any AV interruption*)
- Second-degree AV block (*intermittent* AV conduction)
- Third-degree (or complete) AV block (*complete* interruption of AV conduction)

1.2.8   First-Degree AV Block

PR interval is >200 ms with all P waves conducted to the ventricle; it is most commonly iatrogenic in patients treated with β- and Ca+channel blockers and digoxin or can be secondary to vagal hypertonia; less often the cause is an acute coronary syndrome of the right coronary artery involving AV node [15].

1.2.9   Second-Degree AV Block Type I (Wenckebach: Mobitz I)

There is a progressive increase of the PR interval, until a P wave is not followed by a QRS complex. The block is usually located in the AV node ("suprahisian"). Most common causes are drugs (β- and Ca++ channel blockers, digoxin) and vagal hypertonia. It can also be secondary to ischemia of the AV branch of the right or the circumflex coronary artery. It can rarely evolve to a higher degree AV block. Therefore therapeutic options are based on the identification of the causes and usually require no more than observation. When symptomatic and if vagal tone is involved, atropine 0.5 mg IV bolus (up to 3 mg in total) can transiently improve clinical status.

1.2.10   Higher Degree AV Blocks (Second-Degree AV Block Type II and Third-Degree AV Block)

Advanced AV blocks are a severe condition, which can quickly evolve into hemodynamic instability and/or cardiac arrest.

1.2.11   Second-Degree AV Block Type II (Mobitz II)

One or more P waves are not followed by a QRS complex without a progressive increase of the PR interval. Causes can be drugs (β- and Ca++ channel blockers, digoxin, and other drugs as lithium) or a damage of the conduction pathways. It can be related to an acute coronary syndrome sometimes involving the left anterior descending coronary or one of its septal branches. It may easily evolve to a third-degree block or asystole, so it should be closely monitored.

1.2.12 Third-Degree AV Block

The ECG in the complete AV block shows a complete dissociation between atrial and ventricular activity with the complete absence of any AV conduction. Depending on the level of the block (suprahisian or infrahisian), the QRS morphology and ventricular rate can be different: in suprahisian block, escape rhythm arises from the AV junction (usually at 35–40 bpm, with narrow QRS complex); in infrahisian block, the rhythm arises from the ventricle; rate is less than 30 bpm with wide QRS complex.

In the presence of acute coronary syndrome, suprahisian blocks are usually secondary to an ischemia of the right coronary artery, while infrahisian blocks are frequently due to a huge ischemia within the interventricular septum due to a stenosis/occlusion of the left anterior descending coronary. Suprahisian blocks, like second-degree AV block type I, can be secondary to ischemia of the AV branch of the right or circumflex coronary artery and are usually more benign and recover spontaneously.

Complete AV block may also be related to drugs reducing AV conduction (β- and Ca^{++} channel blockers or digoxin) or reducing intraventricular conduction (as most antiarrhythmic drugs, leading to infrahisian blocks).

1.2.13 Accelerated Idioventricular Rhythm

In the presence of increased automaticity, ventricular rate may be higher than sinus rate (especially in the presence of sinus bradycardia), despite not exceeding 100/min. It is usually benign and asymptomatic; it can be a sign of reperfusion during acute coronary syndromes and should be treated only in presence of significant symptoms or hemodynamic impairment with drugs increasing sinus rate amines and atrial or ventricular pacing.

1.2.14 Treatment:

Treating an advanced-degree AV block requires fast choices [11–13, 16, 17]:

If hemodynamically unstable (Table 1.3):
- Activate the cardiologist for an IV pacing; discuss with him about the value of a coronarography when acute coronary syndrome is likely.
- As soon as possible, start transcutaneous pacing (with sedation).
- If not available, start drugs: dopamine (2–10 mcg/kg/min) or adrenaline (2–10 mcg/min).

Table 1.3 Unstable bradyarrhythmias

Treatment basic points consist in:
ECG, blood pressure, heart rate, respiratory rate, sat O_2 monitoring, hemodynamic assessment
Drugs: atropine, adrenaline or dopamine, isoproterenol
Guarantee the normal hemodynamic state
Emergency pacing should be considered if the need to maintain hemodynamic stability is imminent. As obvious this can be used only as a temporary means to bring the patient to a more stable solution (e.g., IV pacemaker)

If stable:

Evaluate the patient, and collect medical and drugs history; discuss with the cardiologist the management.

1.2.15 Pitfalls

• Confounding third-degree AV block with other bradyarrhythmias, in particular when similar atrial and ventricular rate are present ("iso-rhythmic dissociation"). It is necessary to evaluate very carefully the presence of the P wave (especially in leads V1 and DII) and the correlation with ventricular activity.
• Know your drugs: Atropine is quite ineffective on infrahisian blocks; amines increase oxygen consumption; isoprenaline–isoproterenol may provoke ventricular tachyarrhythmias, so it should be avoided, if possible, in the presence of ischemia.
• Always check if the transcutaneous pacing is achieving consistent capture by checking the femoral pulse.
• A low heart rate may not always be the cause of symptoms; it can be just a sign of other diseases. For example, sinus bradycardia and hypotension may be due to the vagal response in the presence of aortic dissection or Cushing's reflex during intracranial hypertension; in acute renal failure, elevated serum potassium can lead to significant bradyarrhythmias, while dehydration in prerenal acute renal failure can be the cause of the hypotension.

1.2.16 When Should the Consultant Cardiologist Be Called?

Any hemodynamic instability requires immediate intervention and support by the cardiologist to define the underlying causes and to help in the treatment.

High-degree AV blocks should be admitted to a monitoring-capable structure. Drugs withdrawn and indication to permanent pacemaker implantation have to be defined with the cardiologist [13].

A drug-related bradyarrhythmia may resolve after withdrawing the proarrhythmic treatment and requires amines or only temporary pacing.

Not all bradyarrhythmias need to be admitted into a cardiology ward. In the absence of high-degree AV block, stable patients may be safely admitted into medicine ward or even considered for discharge with an outpatient clinic follow-up program [1, 13, 17].

1.2.17 Definitive Pacemaker Indications

Briefly, indications to permanent pacing, in absence of transient or correctable causes, can be summarized as follows [19]:

Alternating or progressive bundle block (right bundle alternating with left bundle, right bundle + left anterior alternating with left posterior fascicular hemiblock)

Second-degree type II AV block: requires pacing when hemodynamically unstable and when the block is located in His bundle or below, even in asymptomatic patients

Third-degree AV block: indicates pacing in all acquired types, associated with syncope, hemodynamic instability, HR <40 bpm, or RR >3000 ms pauses

In older patients it's often difficult to determine the real cost/benefit ratio of a permanent pacemaker, and the balance between conservative and aggressive therapy should be discussed.

Absence of symptoms, a basal heart rate greater than 40 bpm, and the capacity of substitutive rhythm to increase the rate during physical activity may allow an observational strategy instead of a pacing immediate intervention [17].

1.2.18 A Suggested Algorithm/Pathway for Diagnosis and Treatment

All patients	What to do	How to do
	Assess hemodynamic status	Clinical evaluation NIBP, HR, RR, sat O2, body temperature monitoring, IV access
	Identify arrhythmia	ECG
	Identify underlying causes	Medical history, clinical evaluation, ECG, labs, EGA, echocardiography, chest X-ray, expert consulting
	Treat hemodynamic instability	Treat reversible causes; administer appropriate drugs; consider cardioversion or pacing if indicated

Tachyarrhythmia			**What to do**	**How to do**
			Treat instability	Perform immediate cardioversion (with procedural sedation if possible)
			Identify arrhythmia	ECG
	If narrow QRS complex			Manual maneuvers, adenosine if regular, beta-blockers, or Ca++ channel blockers. Consider rhythm control (CVES or drugs) if onset <48 h or rate control ± anticoagulant therapy if >48 h. Consider cardiologist consultant. Admit to ward if poorly tolerated hemodynamic status, severe or evolving underlying pathology, and uncontrolled heart rate regardless initial therapy
	If wide QRS complex			Consider adenosine only if regular monomorphic QRS is present; antiarrhythmic infusion, cardiologist consulting. Admit to ward if evolutive organic cardiopathy, persistence of tachyarrhythmia regardless antiarrhythmic therapy, polymorphic tachycardia, poorly tolerated hemodynamic status

Bradyarrhythmia	**What to do**	**How to do**
	Treat instability	Use atropine, dopamine, adrenaline, or isoprenaline or isoproterenol or perform immediate transthoracic pacing (with procedural sedation if possible). Consult the cardiologist
	Sinus bradycardia	Hemodynamic support, atropine. Identify and treat the underlying causes
	Identify arrhythmia	ECG
	Sick sinus syndrome	Dynamic ECG loop recorder, cardiologist evaluation; consider pacemaker implant
	If First-degree AV block or Second-degree AV block type I	Identify and treat underlying causes. Admit to ward if poorly tolerated hemodynamic status, severe or evolving underlying pathology, uncontrolled heart rate regardless initial therapy
	If high-degree AV blocks (II type II or III)	Be prepared to pace; consult the cardiologist. Admit to a monitoring capable ward

References

1. Neumar RW, Otto CW, Link MS, Kronick SL, Shuster M, Callaway CW, Kudenchuk PJ, Ornato JP, McNally B, Silvers SM, Passman RS, White RD, Hess EP, Tang W, Davis D, Sinz E, Morrison LJ. Adult advanced cardiovascular life support: 2010 American Heart Association Guidelines for Cardiopulmonary Resuscitation and Emergency Cardiovascular Care. Circulation. 2010;122(18):S729–67.
2. Hood RE, Shorofsky SR. Management of arrhythmias in the emergency department. Cardiol Clin. 2006;24:125–33.

3. Delacrétaz E. Supraventricular tachycardia. N Engl J Med. 2006;354:1039–51.
4. Gross JB, Farmington CT, Bailey PL, Rochester NY, Connis RT, Woodinville WA, Cote´ CJ, Chicago IL, Davis FG, Burlington MA, Epstein BS, Washington DC, Gilbertson L, Boston MA, Nickinovich DG, Bellevue WA, Zerwas JM, Houston TX, Zuccaro G, Cleveland OH. Practice guidelines for sedation and analgesia by non-Anesthesiologists: an updated report by The American Society of Anesthesiologists Task Force on Sedation And Analgesia By Non-Anesthesiologists. Anesthesiology. 2002;96:1004–17
5. Tan G, Irwin MG. Recent advances in using propofol by non-anesthesiologists. F1000 Med Rep. 2010 Nov 11,2:79. doi:10.3410/M2-79.
6. Godwin SA, Burton JH, Gerardo CJ, Hatten BW, Mace SE, Silvers SM, Fesmire FM. Procedural sedation and analgesia in the emergency department. Ann Emerg Med. 2014;63:247–58.
7. Link MS. Evaluation and initial treatment of supraventricular tachycardia. N Engl J Med. 2012;367:1438–48.
8. January CT, Wann LS, Alpert JS, Calkins H, Cigarroa JE, Cleveland Jr JC, Conti JB, Ellinor PT, Ezekowitz MD, Field ME, Murray KT, Sacco RL, Stevenson WG, Tchou PJ, Tracy CM, Yancy CW. 2014 AHA/ACC/HRS guideline for the management of patients with atrial fibrillation: a report of the American College of Cardiology/American Heart Association Task Force on Practice Guidelines and the Heart Rhythm Society. J Am Coll Cardiol. 2014;64:e1–76.
9. Oreto G, Luzza F, Satullo G, Donato A, Carbone V, Calabrò MP. Tachicardia a QRS larghi: un problema antico e nuovo. G Ital Cardiol. 2009;10:580–95.
10. Brugada P, Brugada J, Mont L, Smeets J, Andries EW. A new approach to the differential diagnosis of a regular tachycardia with a wide QRS complex. Circulation. 1991;83:1649–59.
11. Grantham HJ. Emergency management of acute cardiac arrhythmias. Aust Fam Physician. 2007;36:492–7.
12. Brady WJ, Harrigan RA. Evaluation and management of bradyarrhythmias in the emergency department. Emerg Med Clin North Am. 1998;16:361–88.
13. Lewalter T, Lickfett L, Schwab JO, Yang A, Lüderitz B. The emergency management of cardiac arrhythmia. Dtsch Arztebl. 2007;104:1172–80.
14. Semelka M, Gera J, Usman S. Sick sinus syndrome: a review. Am Fam Physician. 2013;87: 691–6.
15. Crisel RK, Farzaneh-Far R, Na B, Whooley MA. First-degree atrioventricular block is associated with heart failure and death in persons with stable coronary artery disease: data from the Heart and Soul Study. Eur Heart J. 2011;32:1875–80.
16. Brignole M, Auricchio A, Baron-Esquivias G, Bordachar P, Boriani G, Breithardt OA, et al. 2013 ESC guidelines on cardiac pacing and cardiac resynchronization therapy: the Task Force on cardiac pacing and resynchronization therapy of the European Society of Cardiology (ESC). Developed in collaboration with the European Heart Rhythm Association (EHRA). Eur Heart J. 2013;34:2281–329.
17. Edhag O, Swahn A. Prognosis of patients with complete heart block or arrhythmic syncope who were not treated with artificial pacemakers. A long-term follow-up study of 101 patients. Acta Med Scand. 1976;200:457–63.

Syncope: First Evaluation and Management in the Emergency Department

2

Franco Giada and Andrea Nordio

2.1 Epidemiology of Syncope

Epidemiological studies conducted in the USA have estimated that 30 % of the general population experience at least one episode of syncope in their lifetime [1], which is responsible for about 1–3 % of admissions to the emergency department (ED) and 1–3 % of hospitalizations [2]. In Italy, syncope accounts for 1–2 % of both admissions to the ED and all hospitalizations [3–7]. About half of the patients attending emergency facilities for syncope are subsequently hospitalized; the mean duration of hospitalization is about 8 days [3–7]. Moreover, in industrialized countries the progressive aging of the population, together with the higher prevalence of syncope among elderly subjects, are likely to increase the impact of syncope on healthcare systems in the near future [6].

2.2 Costs of Syncope

The fact that syncope may be caused by pathological conditions that have a severe prognosis, together with the lack of a diagnostic gold standard, results in frequent hospitalization and the prescription of numerous costly instrumental investigations, which increase healthcare costs. One North American study [8] estimated in 1993 that the mean annual cost per patient hospitalized for syncope was US$4132. In the case of recurrent syncope, this figure rose to US$5281. In the USA the total annual

F. Giada (✉)
Cardiovascular Department, P.F. Calvi Hospital,
Via Largo San Giorgio 3, 30033 Noale-Venice, Italy
e-mail: francogiada@hotmail.com

A. Nordio
Cardiovascular Department, Ospedali Riuniti and University of Trieste, Trieste, Italy

© Springer International Publishing Switzerland 2016
M. Zecchin, G. Sinagra (eds.), *The Arrhythmic Patient in the Emergency Department: A Practical Guide for Cardiologists and Emergency Physicians*,
DOI 10.1007/978-3-319-24328-3_2

cost of syncope amounts to \$2.4 billion, similar to that for chronic respiratory diseases and human immunodeficiency virus. In studies conducted in Italy, the mean cost per patient hospitalized for syncope is reported to vary from €1000 to €3000 [9]. These costs are chiefly conditioned by the duration of hospitalization and by the number and type of diagnostic investigations carried out.

Thus, syncope places a considerable burden on healthcare resources. The implementation of an appropriate diagnostic and therapeutic strategy for tackling the problem of syncope in the ED therefore constitutes a challenge from clinical, organizational, and economic standpoints.

2.2.1   Difficulties in the Management of Patients with Syncope in the ED

Syncope is defined as a self-limiting transient loss of consciousness (TLOC), which usually causes falls. The onset of syncope is relatively sudden and the recovery is spontaneous, complete, and rapid. The underlying pathophysiological mechanism is transitory global brain hypoperfusion [10].

The first difficulty encountered in ED in the management of patients who present with TLOC is to distinguish syncope from losses of consciousness (Fig. 2.1) not caused by cerebral hypoperfusion (e.g., epilepsy, metabolic disorders, vertebrobasilar transient ischemic attack, hypoxia), or from conditions with only apparent loss

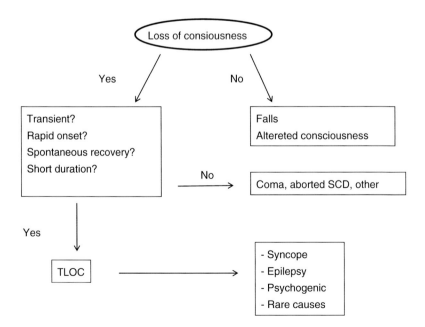

Fig. 2.1   Context of transient loss of consciousness. *SCD* sudden cardiac death, *TLOC* transient loss of consciousness

Table 2.1 Conditions incorrectly diagnosed as syncope	Disorders with partial or complete LOC (without global cerebral hypoperfusion)
	Epilepsy
	Metabolic disorders including hypoglycemia, hypoxia, hyperventilation with hypocapnia
	Intoxication
	Vertebrobasilar TIA
	Disorders without impairment of consciousness
	Cataplexy
	Drop attacks
	Falls
	Functional (psychogenic pseudosyncope)
	TIA of carotid origin

LOC loss of consciousness, *TIA* transient ischemic attack

of consciousness (drop attack, cataplexy, psychogenic pseudosyncope, accidental falls in the elderly) [10] (Table 2.1). Moreover from an etiological standpoint, syncope is classified within three main groups: neuromediated or reflex (representing the epidemiologically prevalent cause of syncope), orthostatic, and cardiac (arrhythmic or structural, the second most common cause of syncope). Each of these groups comprises numerous disorders that may manifest in the form of syncope and are not always easy to evaluate (Table 2.2). Finally, the prognostic significance of syncope depends on the underlying pathology, ranging from the generally benign prognosis seen in neuromediated syncope to the more severe prognosis associated with cardiac syncope.

This syncope often raises diagnostic and therapeutic problems which is proved by the diversity of the pathways followed by patients attending the ED. Indeed, data from the literature [4–7] reveal that these patients may be hospitalized in cardiology, neurology, pediatric, geriatric, internal medicine, and orthopedic wards. These patients then undergo, often inappropriately, several instrumental examinations that are costly and have a low diagnostic yield. The result is that hospitalization is prolonged and healthcare costs rise, while a correct diagnosis of the cause of syncope fails to be reached in a high percentage of cases. As the risk of malpractice suits is high in this field, ED physicians often adopt a strategy of "self-defense," which results in an increase of the number of hospitalizations and inappropriate instrumental investigations. Thus, the current management of syncope displays little diagnostic efficacy and considerable economic inefficiency.

The factors underlying these disappointing results can be summed up as follows: insufficient competence and attention on the part of physicians with regard to the differential diagnosis of TLOC, owing to the difficulty of tackling this problem in a multidisciplinary manner; a "defensive" stance prompted by the possible legal implications of a wrong diagnosis; and, in various healthcare institutions, the lack of diagnostic and therapeutic facilities specialized in the management of syncope patients [11, 12].

Table 2.2 Classification of syncope

Neurally mediated syncope
Vasovagal cause
Mediated by emotional distress (fear, pain, instrumentation blood phobia)
Orthostatic stress
Situational
Sneeze, cough
Gastrointestinal stimulation (defecation, abdominal pain, swallowing)
After micturition
After exercise
Postprandial
Others
Carotid sinus syncope
Forms without apparent triggers or atypical presentation
Orthostatic hypotension syncope
Primary autonomic failure
Pure autonomic failure, multiple atrophy, Parkinson disease with autonomic failure
Lewy body dementia
Secondary autonomic failure
Diabetes, amyloidosis, uremia, spinal injuries
Drug-induced orthostatic hypotension
Alcohol, vasodilators, diuretics, antidepressants
Volume depletion
Hemorrhage, diarrhea, vomiting, etc
Cardiovascular syncope
Arrhythmia as primary cause
Bradycardia: sinus node dysfunction, AV conduction system disease, implanted device dysfunction
Tachycardia: supraventricular, ventricular
Drug-induced bradycardia and arrhythmias
Structural disease
Cardiac: valvular diseases, AMI, hypertrophic cardiomyopathy, etc
Others: acute aortic dissection, pulmonary hypertension, pulmonary embolus

2.2.2 The Recommended Management of Syncope in the ED

Most of the direct cost of syncope is attributable to hospitalization. A proper diagnostic evaluation and prognostic stratification of syncope in the ED should limit hospitalization to patients suffering from heart disease, serious neurological diseases, or severe secondary traumas.

In 2009 the European Society of Cardiology developed guidelines on the management of syncope [10]. This document defined what has become the current standard for the management of patients with TLOC and the most valuable diagnostic pathway, and gave recommendations on indications and interpretation of diagnostic tests with indications for hospitalization and treatment.

According to the guidelines, the cornerstone in syncope management in the ED is the initial clinical evaluation, i.e., history, physical examination, recumbent and orthostatic blood pressure measurement, and electrocardiogram (ECG).

Patients should be interrogated about:

- The circumstances (position and activity of the patient, presence of predisposing factors) and symptoms (nausea, dizziness, palpitations) occurring just before the attack
- Manner of fall (slumping or kneeling over), duration, and whether movements were present during LOC (if witnessed)
- Number, frequency of spells, and age at first episode
- Family history of cardiac disease or sudden death, neurological history, metabolic disorders

Consultation by a cardiologist is indicated when a cardiac cause is suspected or ascertained, particularly in cases of:

- Presence of definite heart disease, family history of sudden death, or channelopathy
- Syncope during exertion or in supine position
- Sudden onset of palpitation prior to the syncope

ECG abnormalities such as intraventricular delay with QRS duration >120 ms, Mobitz II second-degree atrioventricular block, sinoatrial pauses >3 s, nonsustained ventricular tachycardia, preexcitation, long or short QT intervals, Brugada pattern, negative precordial T waves suggestive of right ventricular dysplasia, Q waves suggesting previous myocardial infarction, pacemaker/implantable cardioverter-defibrillator malfunction.

Neurological consultation (Fig. 2.2) is indicated for a nonsyncopal TLOC cause (epilepsy, transient ischemic attack, subclavian steal syndrome, psychogenic pseudosyncope), especially in cases of:

- Presence of aura before the event
- Tonic-clonic movements coinciding with the onset of LOC (and not some seconds later) or hemilateral
- Clear automatisms or tongue biting
- Prolonged confusion after the episode
- Family history of seizures, sleepiness or headache after the event

Specific tests such as neurological investigations or blood tests are only indicated for a suspicion of nonsyncopal TLOC.

This strategy requires adequate clinical competence on the part of all of the physicians involved in the management of these patients. Table 2.3 presents the diagnostic criteria that permit a diagnosis of the causes of syncope in the ED by means of initial evaluation, and Table 2.4 lists the clinical features that suggest a diagnosis.

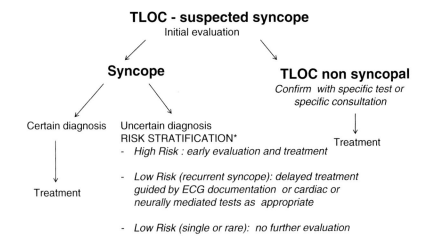

Fig. 2.2 Diagnostic flowchart of patients with suspected T-LOC.*May require laboratory investigations. *ECG* electrocardiographic, *TLOC* transient loss of consciousness

Table 2.3 Diagnostic criteria of causes of syncope with initial evaluation

Vasovagal syncope is diagnosed if syncope is precipitated by emotional distress or orthostatic stress, and is associated with typical prodrome
Situational syncope is diagnosed if syncope occurs during or immediately after specific triggers listed in Table 2.2
Orthostatic syncope is diagnosed when it occurs after standing up and there is documentation of OH
Arrhythmia-related syncope is diagnosed by ECG when there is:
Persistent bradycardia (<40 bpm in awake or repetitive sinoatrial block or sinus pauses >3 s)
Mobitz II or III degree AV block (second or third degree)
Alternating BBB (left and right)
VT or rapid paroxysmal SVT
Polymorphic VT nonsustained and long or short QT interval
PM or ICD malfunction with cardiac pauses
Cardiac ischemia related syncope is diagnosed when syncope presents with ECG evidence of acute ischemia with or without myocardial infarction
Cardiovascular syncope is diagnosed when syncope presents in patients with prolapsing atrial myxoma, severe aortic stenosis, pulmonary hypertension, pulmonary embolus, or acute aortic dissection

AV atrioventricular, *BBB* bundle-branch block, *ECG* electrocardiogram, *PM* pacemaker, *ICD* implantable cardioverter-defibrillator, *OH* orthostatic hypotension, *SVT* supraventricular tachycardia, *VT* ventricular tachycardia, *VVS* vasovagal syncope

The ideal TLOC management should lead, through initial clinical evaluation, to an identification of the nature of the TLOC (syncope or syncope-like conditions) and, in the case of syncope, to an etiological diagnosis and a rapid stratification of patients into three categories (Fig. 2.3):

Table 2.4 Clinical features suggesting a diagnosis at initial evaluation

Neurally mediated syncope
Absence of heart disease
Recurrent syncope history
After sudden unexpected unpleasant sight, sound, smell, pain
Vomiting, nausea during syncope
Prandial or postprandial
After exertion
With head rotation or pressure on carotid sinus
Syncope due to orthostatic hypotension
After standing up
Start or changes of dosage of vasodepressive drugs
Prolonged standing (crowded hot places)
Autonomic neuropathy or Parkinsonism
Standing after exertion
Cardiovascular syncope
Structural heart disease
Family history of channelopathy or USD
Supine or during exertion
ECG findings suggesting arrhythmic syncope:
LBBB or RBBB combined with LA or LP fascicular block
Intraventricular conduction abnormalities (QRS >120 s)
Mobitz I second-degree AV block
Asymptomatic inappropriate sinus bradycardia (<50 bpm)
Nonsustained VT
Preexcited QRS complexes
Long or short QT intervals
Early repolarization
RBBB pattern with ST elevation in leads V1–V3
Q waves suggesting myocardial infarction

USD unexpected sudden death, *LBBB* left bundle-branch block, *RBBB* right bundle-branch block, *LA* left anterior, *LP* left posterior, *VT* ventricular tachycardia

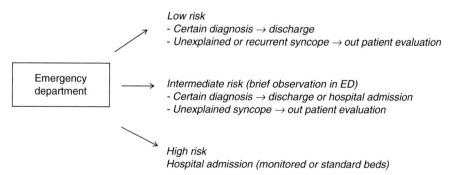

Fig. 2.3 Diagnostic pathway for the management of patients admitted to the ED for syncope

- *Low-risk patients*, who can be handled in the outpatient clinic by the general practitioner or specialist, on an ordinary time schedule, and requiring few, if any, selected examinations [15]; this group includes patients with very likely neurogenic syncope and without injuries
- *Intermediate-risk patients*, who need to be managed within a short time in a specialist outpatient clinic or by means of brief observation in the emergency department, when high risk is not evident but cannot be immediately excluded
- *High-risk patients*, who need to be hospitalized urgently and to immediately undergo appropriate diagnostic and therapeutic procedures. This group includes patients with severe structural or coronary heart disease (heart failure, severe left ventricular dysfunction, previous myocardial infarction), clinical or ECG features suggesting arrhythmic syncope (see above), or important comorbidities (Table 2.5)

Finally, the European guidelines recommend that rapid risk stratification in the ED can be achieved by using the following two scores:

- The OESIL Risk Score [12], which is easy to apply and it includes age >65 years, underlying disease, syncope without prodromes, and an abnormal ECG. A total score of 0 represents 0 % mortality and a score of 1 is associated with <1 % mortality at 1 year. Scores of 3 (mortality of 35 % derivation/29 % validation sets) and 4 (mortality of 57 % and 53 % derivation and validation sets, respectively) carry significantly greater risk.
- The EGSYS Risk Score [13], which shows that the presence of abnormal ECG and/or the presence of structural cardiac disease are the main factors predictive

Table 2.5 Clinical criteria to identify short-term high-risk patients

Severe structural CAD (HF, low LVEF, MI)
Clinical or ECG aspects suggesting arrhythmic syncope
During exertion or supine
Palpitations (during the syncope)
Bifascicular block
Intraventricular conduction abnormalities (QRS >120 ms)
Inadequate sinus bradycardia or SA block in absence of negative chronotropic medications or physical training
Preexcited QRS complex
Prolonged or short QT interval
RBBB pattern with ST elevation (V1–V3 leads)
Negative T waves in right precordial leads, epsilon waves, and ventricular late potentials (ARVC)
Important comorbidities
Anemia (severe)
Electrolyte disturbance

CAD coronary artery disease, *HF* heart failure, *LVEF* left ventricular ejection fraction, *MI* myocardial infarction, *RBBB* right bundle-branch block, *ARVC* arrhythmogenic right ventricular cardiomyopathy

Table 2.6 Risk stratification at initial evaluation in OESIL and EGSYS studies

Study	Risk factors	Score	Endpoints	Results (validation cohort)
OESIL [12]	Abnormal ECG	0–4 (1 point each item)	1 year total mortality	0 % score 0
	Cardiovascular disease (history)			0.6 % score 1
	Lack of prodrome			14 % score 2
	Age >65 years			29 % score 3
EGSYS [13]	Palpitations before syncope (+4)	Sum of + and – points	2 year total mortality	2 % score < 3
	Abnormal ECG and or heart disease (+3)			21 % score ≥3
	Syncope during effort (+3)			
	Syncope while supine (+2)		Cardiac syncope	2 % score < 3
	Predisposing/precipitating factors (−1)			13 % score 3
	Autonomic prodrome (nausea, vomiting) (−1)			33 % score 4
				77 % score > 4

of mortality in 2 years; this score has a very good diagnostic yield in identifying syncope of cardiac origin (Table 2.6).

This strategic course underlines that prognostic stratification and the choice of instrumental investigations selected on the basis of the characteristics of each patient are crucial to the cost-effective management of patients with syncope in the ED [14–17].

References

1. Savage DD, Corwin L, McGee LD, et al. Epidemiology features of isolated syncope: the Framingham study. Stroke. 1985;16:626–9.
2. Day SC, Cook EF, Funkenstain H, Goldman L. Evaluation and outcome of emergency room patients with transient loss of consciousness. Am J Med. 1982;73:15–23.
3. Ammirati F, Colivicchi F, Minardi G, et al. Gestione della sincope in ospedale: lo studio OESIL (Osservatorio Epidemiologico della Sincope nel Lazio). G Ital Cardiol. 1999;29:533–9.
4. Del Greco M, Cozzio S, Scillieri M, Cappari F, Scivales A, Disertori M. The ECSIT study (Epidemiology and Costs of Syncope in Trento). Diagnostic pathway of syncope and analysis of the impact of guidelines in a district general hospital. Ital Heart J. 2003;4:99–106.
5. Haan MN, Selby JV, Quensenberry CP, et al. The impact of aging and chronic disease on use of hospital and outpatient service in a large HMO. J Am Geriat Soc. 1997;45:667–74.

6. Nyman JA, Krahn AD, Bland PC, et al. The costs of recurrent syncope of unknown origin in elderly patients. PACE. 1999;22:1386–94.
7. Olde Nordkamp LAR, van Dijk N, Ganzeboom KS, Reitsma JB, Luitse JSK, Dekker LRC, et al. Syncope prevalence in ED compared to that in the general practice and population: a strong selection process. Am J Emerg Med. 2009;27:271–9.
8. Sun BC, et al. Direct medical costs of syncope-related hospitalizations in the United States. Am J Cardiol. 2005;95(5):668–71.
9. Del Rosso A, Bernadeschi M, Ieri A. Costi sociali della sincope. Ital Heart J Suppl. 2000;1:772–6.
10. The Task Force for the Diagnosis and Management of Syncope of the European Society of Cardiology (ESC). Developed in collaboration with, European Heart Rhythm Association (EHRA), Heart Failure Association (HFA), and Heart Rhythm Society (HRS). Guidelines for the diagnosis and management of syncope. Eur Heart J. 2009;30(21):2631–71.
11. Giada F, Ammirati F, Bartoletti A, Del Rosso A, Dinelli M, Foglia-Manzillo G, et al. La Syncope Unit: un nuovo modello organizzativo per la gestione del paziente con sincope. G Ital Cardiol. 2010;11:323–8.
12. Colivicchi F, Ammirati F, Melina D, Guido V, Imperoli G, Santini M. Development and prospective validation of a risk stratification system for patients with syncope in the emergency department: the OESIL risk score. Eur Heart J. 2003;24:811–9.
13. Del Rosso A, Ungar A, Maggi R, Giada F, Petix NR, De Santo T, et al. Clinical predictors of cardiac syncope at initial evaluation in patients referred urgently to a general hospital: the EGSYS score. Heart. 2009;94:1620–6.
14. Shen WK, Decker WW, Smars PA, Goyal DG, Walker AE, Hodge DO, et al. Syncope evaluation in the emergency department study (SEEDS). A multidisciplinary approach to syncope management. Circulation. 2004;110:3636–45.
15. Brignole M, Disertori M, Menozzi C, et al. The management of syncope referred for emergency to general hospitals with and without Syncope Unit facility. Europace. 2003;5:293–8.
16. Disertori M, Brignole M, Menozzi C, et al. Management of syncope referred for emergency to general hospitals. Europace. 2003;5:283–91.
17. Brignole M, Menozzi C, Bartoletti A, Giada F, Lagi A, Ungar A, et al. A new management of syncope: prospective systematic guideline-based evaluation of patients referred urgently to general hospitals. Eur Heart J. 2006;27:76–82.

Management of Bradyarrhythmias in Emergency

3

Luca Salvatore, Silvia Magnani, Gerardina Lardieri, and Elena Zambon

The sudden appearance in patients of changes in heart rhythm is a situation that requires rapid diagnosis and treatment in emergency departments and intensive care units. The slowdown and block of cardiac impulse conduction form the basis of symptomatic bradycardia.

The prevalence of cardiac bradyarrhythmias and conduction disturbances in outpatients evaluated for the first time is 30–40 %, with an incidence of 3 % for atrioventricular (AV) block and sinus node dysfunction, and 8 % for disorders of intraventricular conduction [1].

Dysfunction of the sinus node has significant clinical implications. Development of concomitant AV block is not uncommon (incidence 8.4 %), as is the presence or appearance of atrial fibrillation (AF), especially in patients already treated with only ventricular pacing (incidence 22 %), with a consequent high risk of systemic thromboembolism [2, 3]. In elderly patients a low heart rate can promote the development or worsening of heart failure, even in the presence of preserved systolic function [4].

The onset of arrhythmias after cardiac and noncardiac surgery, a relatively common occurrence, is a major predictor of morbidity of surgical procedures and is associated with a prolonged hospital stay, although severe bradyarrhythmias requiring treatment occur in less than 1 % of cases. Triggers are generally transient events such as hypoxia, myocardial ischemia, excess catecholamine, or electrolyte disorders [5, 6].

L. Salvatore (✉) • S. Magnani • G. Lardieri • E. Zambon
Cardiovascular Department, Ospedali Riuniti and University of Trieste, Trieste, Italy
e-mail: lucasalvatore@alice.it

© Springer International Publishing Switzerland 2016
M. Zecchin, G. Sinagra (eds.), *The Arrhythmic Patient in the Emergency Department: A Practical Guide for Cardiologists and Emergency Physicians*, DOI 10.1007/978-3-319-24328-3_3

3.1   Anatomy and Pathophysiology

The cardiac impulse begins in the *sinus atrial node*, located in the upper lateral wall of the right atrium near the superior vena cava, vascularized by the right coronary artery (60 %) and the circumflex artery (40 %). The impulse reaches the AV node, which, through the nodal-Hisian system, connects the atria with the ventricles. The nodal-Hisian system is formed by the *AV node* (located in the front part of the Koch triangle, vascularized by the right coronary artery) and the *bundle of His* (vascularized by both the left and right coronary artery). The bundle of His is divided into the *right branch* (vascularized by the anterior descending artery and right coronary artery) and the *left branch*, which in turn is divided into two bundles, the anterior (vascularized by the anterior descending artery) and the posterior (vascularized by the circumflex artery). From here the Purkinje fibers originate, guaranteeing simultaneous activation of the ventricles.

3.2   Bradycardia

A heart rate of less than 60 bpm is usually considered as bradycardia. The usual symptoms of bradycardia are asthenia, fatigue, dyspnea, chest discomfort or pain, prior or complete loss of consciousness, light-headedness, and decreased level of consciousness. Frequent noticeable signs include hypotension and/or orthostatic hypotension, diaphoresis, bradycardia-related (escape) frequent premature ventricular complexes, or other ventricular tachyarrhythmias. Usually the symptoms are relevant when the heart rate is lower than 40 bpm, or higher in the presence of a pre- or coexistent cardiac disease.

Hemodynamically unstable bradycardia may represent a serious life-threatening emergency, with 30-day mortality rates of up to 16 % being reported [7–9]. Bradycardia can be the expression of the dysfunction of *automaticity* or the *conduction* of the electrical impulse, and can be detected at all levels of the conduction system (sinoatrial node, AV node, intraventricular branches).

3.3   Sinus Node Dysfunction

The main manifestations of sinus node dysfunction are *sinus bradycardia* and *sinus arrest*.

Sinus node dysfunction recognizes *intrinsic* causes: degenerative disease, chronic or acute ischemia, infiltrative disease (amyloidosis, hemochromatosis, tumors), inflammatory causes (pericarditis, myocarditis), musculoskeletal disease (Duchenne dystrophy, Friedreich ataxia), vasculitis (systemic lupus erythematosus, scleroderma), and surgical (atrial septal defect correction); and *extrinsic* causes: drugs (amiodarone, flecainide, propafenone, sotalol, chinidina, disopyramide, procainamide), electrolyte disorders (hyperkalemia), endocrinopathies (hypothyroidism), vagal reflex during ischemia, neuromediated syndrome (vasovagal, cough, carotid sinus hypersensitivity), intracranial hypertension, and obstructive jaundice.

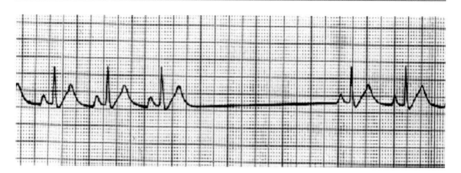

Fig. 3.1 Sinus arrest

3.3.1 Sinus Bradycardia

Sinus bradycardia can be secondary to intrinsic factors such as fibrosis (aging or loss of "pacing cells" [10, 11] resulting from inferior myocardial infarction, or to extrinsic factors such as an increased vagal tone, an abnormal neurocardiogenic reflex, drugs such as β-blockers or Ca^{2+} antagonists, or drugs reducing sympathetic tone such as sympatholytic antihypertensives [12].

The electrocardiogram (ECG) shows a regular sinus rhythm with heart rate lower than 60 bpm and a constant 1:1 AV conduction, with a normal PR interval (120–200 ms); P waves are regular, with the same shape and axis between 0° and 90°.

Symptoms can be absent at rest and may appear only during effort. In general, sinus bradycardia does not require treatment; intravenous atropine can be effective, but is useful only for short-term treatment because of its short half-life; sometimes temporary or permanent pacing may be necessary, favoring atrial over ventricular stimulation [13, 14].

3.3.2 Sinus Arrest

Sinus arrest is the absence of onset of spontaneous atrial impulse. It is generally considered significant when this pause lasts longer than 3 s. The most common causes are tissue fibrosis, ischemia, digoxin intoxication, cerebral ischemia, and excessive vagal tone (Fig. 3.1).

3.4 Atrioventricular Block

Atrioventricular block occurs when the conduction of the atrial impulse to the ventricles slows down or is blocked (paroxysmal or permanently), even though the AV junction is not physiologically refractory.

In the presence of a high atrial rate (e.g., atrial tachycardia or AF), the term AV block is correct only if the ventricular rate is lower than 60 bpm.

There are three anatomical sites of block: (1) above Hisian (inside the AV node), (2) intra-Hisian (inside the His bundle), and (3) infra-Hisian (distal His bundle or bundle branches).

The identification of anatomical site is relevant, as the distal blocks are those with the worst prognosis.

3.4.1 First-Degree AV Block

Every single atrial impulse is followed by a QRS complex, but the PR interval is greater than 200 ms. The block is usually above the AV node, even if there may be a wide QRS complex caused by a coexisting bundle-branch block. In general it is not associated with heart disease, and is usually secondary to increased vagal tone or is drug related (β-blocker or digoxin), although sometimes it can be associated with myocardial ischemia, infiltrative myocardiopathies, myocarditis, Addison disease, or congenital heart disease (septal defect, Ebstein). Prognosis, however, is benign, and no treatment is required. An exception can be the occurrence of a first-degree AV block in aortic valve endocarditis resulting from an abscess of the interventricular septum.

3.4.2 Second-Degree AV Block

Conduction from the atria to the ventricles is intermittent. There are two types of second-degree AV block.

Type I, also known as Mobitz I or Luciani-Wenckebach, involves progressive increase of the PR interval and consequent shortening of the RR interval until a nonconducted P wave develops. The morphology of the QRS complex is normal. The site of the block is usually at or above the AV node [15]. Etiology mainly includes digoxin intoxication, myocardial ischemia (inferior myocardial infarction), excess calcium deposits such as occur in aortic stenosis, or renal insufficiency. It can be also observed in both trained athletes and normal persons during sleep, attributable to increased vagal tone [16–18]. Prognosis is excellent if asymptomatic, while the onset of symptoms such as syncope or heart failure may require the placement of a definitive pacemaker.

Type II (Mobitz II) shows a sudden block of a P wave with a ratio of 3:2, 4:3, and so forth. PP and RR intervals are regular (Fig. 3.2). The block is intra- or infra-Hisian, and tends to progress toward complete AV block with prolonged ventricular pause and syncope [19]. Guidelines favor permanent pacing even in asymptomatic patients with type II block [20].

3.4.3 Atrioventricular Block with 2:1 Conduction

This condition is characterized by an intermittent block with a P/QRS ratio of 2:1, thus having features of both Mobitz I and II. Block can be at any nodal site and

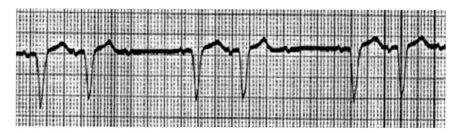

Fig. 3.2 II degree–Mobitz 2 AV block (with intraventricular delay)

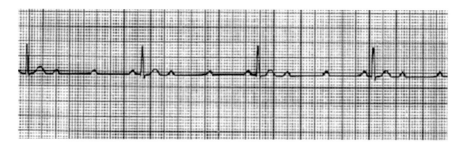

Fig. 3.3 Advanced (3:1) tipo II AV block

intra- or infra-Hisian, the severity depending on the resultant ventricular rate. In an asymptomatic patient a 2:1 block with a coexisting bundle-branch block is an indication for pacing, assuming that the block is infranodal [21].

3.4.4 Advanced AV Block

In advanced AV block, two or more consecutive P waves are blocked with a P/QRS ratio of 3:1, 4:1, and so forth (Fig. 3.3). In everyday practice this term is also used for low-rate permanent AF.

3.4.5 Low-Rate Atrial Fibrillation

The absence of recognizable P wave, irregular RR intervals, and narrow or wide QRS complexes characterizes low-rate AF. Causes are usually drugs (antiarrhythmic, digoxin, β-blockers, Ca^{2+} antagonists), especially in elderly patients with impaired renal and/or liver function, vagal hypertone (young subjects), or impaired AV conduction.

Treatment consists in ensuring hemodynamic normality using drugs (atropine followed by amines) or transcutaneous or transvenous pacing in symptomatic bradycardia.

3.4.6   Third-Degree AV Block

The inability of P waves to conduct to the ventricles (complete block of AV conduction) characterizes third-degree AV block. There is no relationship between P waves and QRS complexes, which are escape beats. Narrow QRS escape rhythms, with regular RR and a frequency between 40 and 60 bpm, are secondary to blocks within the AV node. Wide QRS escape rhythms with frequency between 40 and 20 bpm are secondary to infra-Hisian blocks.

In patients with AF and complete AV block a regular ventricular rate is observed, because of junctional (usually at about 35 bpm) or infra-Hisian escape rhythm.

Third-degree AV block can be secondary to pharmacologic treatments (digoxin, β-blockers, Ca^{2+} antagonists, quinidine, procainamide) or sclerodegenerative phenomena of conduction fibers, or may occur during the acute phase of myocardial infarction. Prognosis is more favorable if associated with inferior myocardial infarction (supra-Hisian block, narrow QRS escape rhythm, and generally spontaneous resolution), while the prognosis is worse in anterior myocardial infarction (infra-Hisian block and wide QRS escape rhythm, generally associated with a wider area and less reversibility of ischemic injury).

Less common causes include infectious diseases (myocarditis, Lyme disease, Chagas disease), rheumatic etiology (Reiter syndrome, scleroderma, rheumatoid arthritis), infiltrative disease (amyloidosis, sarcoidosis, multiple myeloma), electrolyte disorders, and iatrogenic factors (cardiac surgery, radiofrequency ablation) (Fig. 3.4).

3.4.7   Interventricular Block

Left bundle-branch block (LBBB) is a rare finding in the young population, and when present should raise the suspicion of an underlying heart disease. Incidence increases with age [22] and is associated with various causes of heart disease (hypertensive, ischemic, valvular, idiopathic dilated cardiomyopathy). Prognosis depends on the severity of the underlying disease.

Left anterior hemi-block (LAHB), more frequent in the adult male population, is associated with hypertension and ischemic heart disease. Progression to LBBB or complete AV block is uncommon [23].

Left posterior hemi-block (LPHB) is a rare isolated finding because of both the short course and double vascularization of the left posterior fascicle.

Right bundle-branch block (RBBB) as an incidental ECG finding is not often linked to heart disease, but may be associated with systemic hypertension, pulmonary heart disease, or ischemic heart disease.

Bifascicular block commonly indicates the association of an interruption or delay in impulse conduction along both sets of left bundle branch, or along the right branch and one of the two sets of left bundle branch.

RBBB + LAHB, a more common condition, shows a progression to complete AV block in less than 6 % of patients, while RBBB + LPHB, less frequent, has a greater progression toward complete AV block (close to 75 %).

Patients with bifascicular block associated with first-degree AV block (especially infranodal, when the HV interval, documented during invasive electrophysiological evaluation, is >100 ms) have a higher risk for developing complete AV block, and some authors recommend permanent cardiac stimulation [24]. The diagnosis of trifascicular block can be made on surface ECG only in the presence of alternating bundle-branch block (LBBB alternating with RBBB, or RBBB + LAHB alternating with RBBB + LPHB).

3.4.8 Atrioventricular Dissociation

AV dissociation is present when atrial activity is independent from ventricular activity, both occurring at regular rates. AV dissociation is not synonymous with AV block; in fact while patients with AV block also have an AV dissociation, patients with AV dissociation may not have an AV block, for example when an escape junctional (or ventricular) rate is higher than the sinus rate in the absence of retrograde ventricular-atrial conduction.

Elderly patients with degenerative cardiac disease are more likely to have AV dissociation [25].

Treatment depends on the causes, and ranges from antiarrhythmic drug treatment to permanent pacemaker placement.

3.4.9 Conduction Disturbances during Acute Myocardial Infarction

Sinus node dysfunction in the course of myocardial infarction may be secondary to the occlusion of the circumflex artery or the right coronary artery. The bradycardia that follows may favor escape rhythms with narrow QRS, which originate at the junction or in the His bundle and have a heart rate of about 50–60 bpm becoming stable over time, whereas escape rhythms with wide QRS originate from the Purkinje fibers with a heart rate below 40 bpm, are less stable, and may evolve to asystole. The AV block that occurs in the early stages of myocardial infarction is generally secondary to hypervagotonia and is reversible with atropine, while blocks occurring later are frequently related to ischemia of the AV node.

Second-degree type I AV block during inferior myocardial infarction tends to resolve spontaneously within 48 h and does not require invasive treatment unless there is hemodynamic compromise.

Second-degree type II AV block is more likely to progress to complete AV block, and occurs more frequently in anterior myocardial infarction, although it can also occur in inferior myocardial infarction because of occlusion of a large posterior descending artery.

Complete AV block, which is present in 8–13 % of patients with myocardial infarction, occurs in both inferior and anterior myocardial infarction, and can be preceded by fascicular blocks or bundle-branch block with second-degree AV block.

It is associated with a higher incidence of ventricular fibrillation/tachycardia, pulmonary edema, and in-hospital mortality [26].

3.4.10 Cardiac Arrest and Sudden Cardiac Death

The incidence of sudden cardiac death (occuring within 1 h from the onset of cardiac symptoms) is variable, depending on the varying prevalence of coronary disease in different countries [27]. In the USA there are 300,000 cardiac deaths annually, with a total annual incidence of 1 in 1,000 individuals [28].

Ventricular fibrillation is the first rhythm detected in 75–80 % of cases, while in the remaining 20–25 % extreme bradycardia or pulseless electrical activity are causes of cardiac arrest.

Bradyarrhythmic cardiac arrest is secondary to the inability of cardiac automatism to emerge and replace the sinus node or normal function of the AV junction.

Cardiac arrest is more common in advanced cardiac disease, generally as a consequence of extracellular potassium accumulation (secondary to hypoxemia, acidosis, shock, or renal insufficiency), which reduces myocellular automatism.

Pulseless electrical activity is an electrical stable cardiac rhythm in the absence of any effective myocardial contraction. The *primary form* is generally the terminal event of a severe cardiopathy or expression of acute myocardial ischemia, and the *secondary form* is a severe expression of a sudden failure in venous return, such as in pulmonary embolism, cardiac tamponade, or acute cardiac prosthetic valve dysfunction.

Reversible causes such as hypovolemia, hypoxia, cardiac tamponade, pneumothorax, acidosis, and hyperkalemia must be detected and corrected. Pharmacological support involves the use of intravenous epinephrine or atropine (the latter, however, is not effective in infra-Hisian AV block).

External cardiac pacing can be useful, although "asystolic" patients still have a poorer prognosis, regardless of the effectiveness of the stimulation [29].

3.5   Treatment

Sinus node dysfunction generally does not require treatment if asymptomatic. When needed, parasympatholytic drugs (atropine 0.5 mg intravenously, repeatable) can acutely increase the automaticity of the sinus node and improve sinus atrial conduction. Sympathomimetic drugs (theophylline per os) are less frequently used for long-term treatment because of their low efficacy and frequent side effects.

If there is any hemodynamic compromise, such as during an inferior myocardial infarction with right ventricle involvement, temporary endocardial pacing is preferred.

The presence of low cardiac output or heart failure, secondary to bradycardia, should be treated with permanent cardiac stimulation, preferably of the right atrium, to allow the spontaneous maintenance of AV conduction and avoid ventricular stimulation.

Supra-Hisian II AV block generally acutely responds to vagolytic drugs. As mentioned earlier, these drugs should be used with caution in suspected infra-Hisian blocks, which can be exacerbated by the increased cardiac rate and supra-Hisian conduction.

Sympathomimetic drugs such as isoproterenol, which are able to increase the automatism of ventricular "pacemaker subsidiary," can be used in the short term regardless of the level of AV block, in particular when it is likely that the block can be transient or if a temporary pacemaker cannot be immediately applied.

In third-degree AV block vagolytic drugs are not particularly effective, especially in the presence of infra-Hisian block, while sympathomimetic drugs provide valuable support in the acute phase while awaiting a permanent pacemaker.

3.5.1 Temporary Pacemaker

Temporary cardiac pacing is used acutely for critically ill patients who require immediate treatment, and sometimes in noncritical situations when patients are at high risk of developing advanced blocks or cardiac arrest.

An intracardiac approach is usually preferred, generally through the internal jugular vein, the subclavian vein, or the femoral vein.

Transcutaneous pacing, despite not having shown a significant benefit in patients with cardiac arrest [29], may be beneficial for the treatment of severe bradycardia as a "bridge" to a permanent pacemaker.

The main indication remains hemodynamically unstable acute myocardial infarction (Table 3.1). Drug treatment with digitalis, quinidine, class 1C antiarrhythmics, β-blockers, and some calcium antagonists can inhibit sinus node automatism up to the development of severe bradycardia, requiring, if associated with signs and symptoms of hemodynamic compromise, temporary pacing to allow pharmacological washout in safety [30].

Hypervagotonia can occur in carotid sinus hypersensitivity, in pharyngeal or gastroesophageal handling during intubation and/or endoscopy, and with parasympathomimetic or sympatholytic drugs. It is associated with three types of clinical response: the first, or cardioinhibitory, with hemodynamically significant bradyarrhythmia; the second, vasodepressor, with hypotension by peripheral vasodilation; and the third, which is a combination of the first two forms. Sometimes temporary pacing can be useful in intensive care, although these clinical situations are easily reversible with atropine [31].

Myocarditis can require temporary pacing because of transient involvement of the ventricular conduction system.

Complications of temporary pacing include capture failure caused by electrode dislocation (25 %), ventricular tachyarrhythmia related to local irritation of the electrode (10 %), pericarditis (5 %), and cardiac tamponade secondary to right atrium perforation (1 %).

Complications related to central venous access are air embolism (1 %), arterial trauma (1.2 %), pneumothorax (1 %), phlebitis (5.1 %), venous thrombosis (18-34 %), and bacteremia (50 %), although infection of the electrode is low [31].

Table 3.1 Therapeutic approach in conduction disturbances

Sinus atrial dysfunction	Asymptomatic patient: observation Symptomatic patient: atropine 0.5 mg iv repeatable up to 2 mg temporary/permanent pacemaker

AV block	First-degree AV block: observation
	Second-degree AV block
	  Type I asymptomatic: observation symptomatic – atropine 0.5 mg iv repeatable up to 2 mg
	  Type II asymptomatic (advanced or Mobitz 2) or symptomatic → pacemaker implantation
	  narrow QRS → atropine, if ineffective → pacemaker
	  wide QRS → PM implantation
	Third-degree AV block a/symptomatic:
	  narrow QRS → atropine, if ineffective → pacemaker
	  wide QRS → PM implantation

AV block during myocardial infarction	Inferior myocardial infarction
	  First-degree AV block → observation
	  Second-degree AV block:
	    Type I → atropine, if ineffective → temporary pacemaker
	    Type II → temporary pacemaker
	    Third-degree AV block → atropine, if ineffective → temporary pacemaker
	Anterior myocardial infarction:
	  First-degree AV block → observation
	  Second-degree AV block
	    Type I atropine, if ineffective → temporary pacemaker
	    Type II → temporary pacemaker
	    Third-degree AV block → temporary pacemaker

3.5.2 Permanent Pacemaker

Sinus node dysfunction is a major reason for pacemaker implantation (about 46 % of implanted devices) [32] and has a long natural history with a good prognosis in the early stages, although with the progress of the disease and the appearance of symptoms the prognosis becomes less favorable [33].

Atrial pacing is preferable to ventricular pacing alone, although the advantage is reduced in the presence of thromboembolic events or the occurrence of AF [14, 34].

AV block is the second leading cause of pacemaker implantation. Permanent cardiac pacing has improved survival in patients with complete or advanced AV block, particularly if associated with symptoms (syncope or hemodynamic compromise) or in the presence of heart disease [35].

Asymptomatic first- and second-degree (type I) AV blocks do not require permanent cardiac pacing.

Symptomatic or second-degree AV block with slow escape rhythm (type I) and asymptomatic type II block are class II indications for permanent pacemaker implantation.

Complete or advanced AV block (both asymptomatic and symptomatic) and second-degree (type II) AV block, regardless of the level of block, are class I indications for a permanent pacemaker.

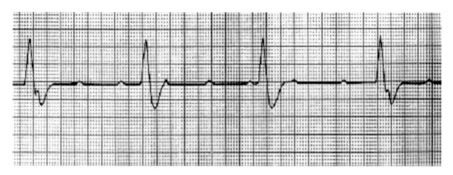

Fig. 3.4 III degree AV block with wide QRS (infra-hisian) escape

Care should be taken in cases of reversible AV block.

Survival in patients with complete AV block not treated with pacemaker implantation is 60 % at 1 year and 30 % at 5 years [35]. Patients treated with permanent pacemakers have been shown to have a 1-year survival comparable with that of the general population [36].

European and American guidelines for Pacemaker implantation [37, 38]
Class I indications
Sinus node dysfunction
Symptomatic sinus bradycardia or chronotropic incompetence
AV block
Second-degree AV block type II
Advanced AV block during sinus rhythm or AF
Complete AV block
Intraventricular block
Trifascicular block (RBBB alternating with LBBB, RBBB+LAHB alternating with RBBB+LPHB)
Bifascicular block (LBBB, RBBB+LAHB, RBBB+LPHB) and second-degree type II or third-degree AV block

Bibliography

1. Vàzquez Ruiz de Castroviejo E, Munoz Bellino J, Lozano Cabezas C, et al. Analysis of the frequency of cardiac arrhythmias and conduction disturbances from a health-care perspective. Rev Esp Cardiol. 2005;58(6):657–65.
2. Sutton R, Kenny RA. The natural history of sinus sick syndrome. Pacing Clin Electrophysiol. 1986;9(6):1110–4.
3. Mandel WJ, Jordan JL, Karagueuzian HS. Disorders of sinus function. Curr Treat Options Cardiovasc Med. 1999;1:179–86.
4. Alboni P, Brignole M, Menozzi C, Scarfò S. Is sinus bradycardia a factor facilitating overt heart failure? Eur Heart J. 1999;20:252–5.

 5. Amar D. Strategies for perioperative arrhythmias. Best Pract Res Clin Anaesthesiol. 2004;18(4):565–77.
 6. Heintz KM, Hollenberg SM. Perioperative cardiac issues: postoperative arrhythmias. Surg Clin North Am. 2005;85(6):1103–14.
 7. Swart G, Brady Jr WJ, DeBehnke DJ, Ma OJ, Aufderheide TP. Acute myocardial infarction complicated by hemodynamically unstable bradyarrhythmia: prehospital and ED treatment with atropine. Am J Emerg Med. 1999;17:647–52.
 8. Brady WJ, Swart G, DeBehnke DJ, Ma OJ, Aufderheide TP. The efficacy of atropine in the treatment of hemodynamically unstable bradycardia and atrioventricular block: prehospital and emergency department considerations. Resuscitation. 1999;41:47–55.
 9. Schwartz B, Vermeulen MJ, Idestrup C, Datta P. Clinical variables associated with mortality in out-of-hospital patients with hemodynamically significant bradycardia. Acad Emerg Med. 2004;11:656–61; Delise P. ARITMIE. C.E.S.I. srl; 2004.
10. Demoulin JC, Kulbertus HE. Histopathological correlates of sick sino-atrial disease. Br Heart J. 1978;40:1384.
11. Shaw DB, Linker NJ, Heaver PA, Evans R. Chronic sinoatrial disorder (sick sinus syndrome): a possible result of cardiac ischemia. Br Heart J. 1987;58:598.
12. Oreto G. riconoscimento del blocco seno atriale di I grado all' elettrocardiogramma standard. G Ital Cardiol. 1982;12:762–6.
13. Rosenquist M, Brandt J, Schuller H. Atrial versus ventricular pacing in sinus node disease: a treatment comparison study. Am Heart J. 1986;111:292.
14. Andersen HR, Nielsen JC, Thomen PE, et al. Long term follow-up of patients from a randomised trial of atrial versus ventricular pacing for sick-sinus syndrome. Lancet. 1997;350:1210–6.
15. Zipes DP. Second degree atrioventricular block. Circulation. 1979;60:465–72.
16. Braunwald E, Zipes DP, Libby P, editors. Heart disease: a textbook of cardiovascular medicine. 6th ed. Philadelphia: WB Saunders; 2001.
17. Strasberg B, Amat-Y-Leon F, Dhingra RC, et al. Natural history of chronic second-degree atrioventricular nodal block. Circulation. 1981;63:1043–9.
18. Meytes I, Kaplinsky E, Yahini JH, Hanne-Paparo N, Neufeld HN. Wenckebach A-V block: a frequent feature following heavy physical training. Am Heart J. 1975;90:426–30.
19. Schweitzer P, Mark H. The effect of atropine on cardiac arrhythmias and conduction. Am Heart J. 1980;100:225–61.
20. Lee TH. Use of cardiac pacemakers and antiarrhythmic devices: ACC/AHA guidelines summary. In: Braunwald E, Zipes DP, Libby P, editors. Heart disease: a textbook of cardiovascular medicine. 6th ed. Philadelphia: WB Saunders; 2001. p. 810–4.
21. Kusomoto FM, Goldschlager N. Cardiac pacing. N Engl J Med. 1996;334:89–98.
22. Siegman-Igra Y, Yahini JH, Goldbourt U. Intraventricular conduction disturbances: a review of prevalence, etiology, and progression for 10 years within a stable population of Israeli adult males. Am Heart J. 1978;96:669.
23. Rowland E. SA node dysfunction, AV block and intraventricular conduction disturbances. Eur Heart J. 1992;13(Suppl H):130–5.
24. Scheinman MM, Peters RW, Modin G, et al. Prognostic value of infranodal conduction time in patients with chronic bundle branch block. Circulation. 1977;56:240–4.
25. Harrigan RA, Perron AD, Brady WJ. Atrioventricular dissociation. Am J Emerg Med. 2001;19:218–22.
26. Clemmensen P, Bates ER, Califf RM. Complete atrioventricular block complicating inferior wall acute myocardial infarction treated with reperfusion therapy. Am J Cardiol. 1991;67:225–30.
27. Priori SG, Aliot E, Blomstrom-Lundqvist C. Task Force on Sudden Cardiac Death of the European Society of Cardiology. Europace. 2002;4:3–18.
28. Myerburg RJ, Kessler KM, Castellanos A. Sudden cardiac death: epidemiology, transient risk, and intervention assessment. Ann Intern Med. 1993;119(12):1187–97.

29. Cummins RO, Graves JR, Larsen MP. Out-of-hospital transcutaneous pacing by emergency medical technicians in patients with asystolic cardiac arrest. N Engl J Med. 1993;328(19):1377–82.
30. Alpert MA, Flaker GC. Arrhythmias associated with sinus node disease. Circulation. 1971;43:836–44.
31. Silver M, Goldschlager N. Temporary transvenous cardiac pacing in the critical care setting. Chest. 1988;93(3):607–13.
32. Elmqvist R. Review of early pacemaker development. Pacing Clin Electrophysiol. 1978;1:535–6.
33. Mond HG, Irwin M, Morillo C, et al. The world survey of cardiac pacing and cardioconvertor defibrillators: calendar 2001. Pacing Clin Electrophysiol. 2004;27:955–64.
34. Lamas GA, Lee KL, Sweeney MO, et al. Ventricular pacing or dual chamber pacing for sinus node dysfunction. N Engl J Med. 2002;346:1854–62.
35. Edhag O, Swahn A. Prognosis of patients with complete heart block or arrhythmic syncope who were not treated with artificial pacemakers. A long term follow up study of 101 patients. Acta Med Scand. 1976;200:457–63.
36. Edhag O. Long term cardiac pacing: experience of fixed rate pacing with an endocardial electrode in 260 patients. Acta Med Scand. 1969;502:64.
37. Brignole M, et al. ESC guidelines on cardiac pacing and cardiac resynchronization therapy. Eur Heart J. 2013; doi:10.1093/eurheartj/eht150.
38. Epstein EE, et al. ACC/AHA/HRS 2008 guidelines for device-based therapy of cardiac rhythm abnormalities. J Am Coll Cardiol. 2008; doi:10.1016/j.jacc.2008.02.032.

Supraventricular Arrhythmias in Emergency

4

Elisabetta Bianco, Marco Bobbo, and Davide Stolfo

The term "supraventricular tachycardia" refers to arrhythmias requiring atrial or atrioventricular nodal tissue, or both, for their initiation and maintenance. Supraventricular tachycardias are often recurrent, occasionally persistent, and a frequent cause of visits to emergency departments (ED) [1].

The following chapter is organized in two main sections dedicated to physician working in ER and cardiologist in order to discuss arguments related to each specific expertise so that patients can receive assessment and treatment personalized on global clinical condition, not only on arrhythmia, in the ED.

4.1   What Physicians Working in ED Should Know

- Timing and modality to treat arrhythmias depends on patient's hemodynamic condition.
- Hemodynamic instability imposes emergent treatment with electrical cardioversion before diagnosis.
- In case of hemodynamic stability it is possible to think about diagnosis and choose best treatment.
- Hemodynamic instability depends on heart rate and on patients' features as age, underlying cardiomyopathy or chronic therapies, electrolyte disturbance, hyperthyroidism, hyperthermia, and drugs intoxication rather than on the type of arrhythmia [2, 3].

E. Bianco
Cardiovascular Department, Cattinara University Hospital, Trieste, Italy
e-mail: elisabetta.bianco@aots.sanita.fvg.it

M. Bobbo • D. Stolfo
Cardiovascular Department, Cattinara University Hospital, Trieste, Italy

© Springer International Publishing Switzerland 2016

43

M. Zecchin, G. Sinagra (eds.), *The Arrhythmic Patient in the Emergency Department: A Practical Guide for Cardiologists and Emergency Physicians*,
DOI 10.1007/978-3-319-24328-3_4

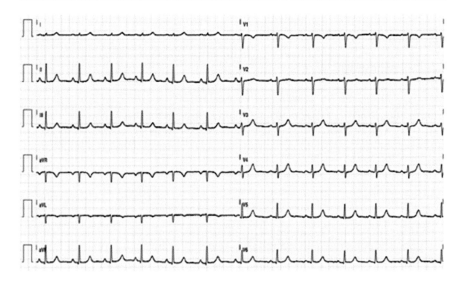

Fig. 4.1 ECG in normal sinus rhythm; with usual setting (paper speed 25 mm/s) 1 mm equals with 40 ms interval

Supraventricular arrhythmias are [4]:

1. Sinus tachycardia
2. Atrial flutter (typical or atypical)
3. Atrial fibrillation (AF)
4. Atrioventricular nodal reentrant tachycardia (AVNRT)
5. Atrioventricular reciprocating tachycardia (AVRT)
6. Atrial/junctional tachycardia (AT)

ECG during arrhythmias differs from normal ECG observed in sinus rhythm. So, first of all, normal ECG must be known [5, 6] (Fig. 4.1):

- Each QRS complex is preceded by a *P wave* with a rate between 60 and 100 bpm with the exception of newborns and infants in whom normal HR is higher (150–230 bpm in newborn) [7].
- P wave is positive in leads I–II and aVL–aVF and in precordial leads from V2–3 to V6, is negative in aVR and can be negative in III, and is biphasic in V1–V2; P wave lasts 120 ms (3 mm).
- Between P wave and QRS complex, there is an isoelectric region (flat line on ECG) which lasts 120–200 ms: the *PR interval*.
- *QRS is narrow* (<110 ms).

While approaching a patient with symptomatic supraventricular tachycardia, physicians must evaluate the patient's clinical status to identify potential reversible causes of tachycardia and to assess the degree of instability and understand if it is related to the tachycardia itself.

Arterial blood pressure, oxygen saturation, electrolyte, and hemoglobin must be evaluated; ECG monitoring and intravenous access must be established.

If possible a 12-lead ECG should be performed during the arrhythmia (and after its interruption) [2].

4.1.1 Patients in Unstable Condition

If the patient demonstrates rate-related cardiovascular compromise with signs and symptoms such as acute altered mental status, ischemic chest discomfort, acute heart failure, hypotension, or other signs of shock suspected to be due to a tachyarrhythmia, proceed to immediate synchronized electrical cardioversion (after sedation of the patient if conscious); provide oxygen if oxygen saturation is below 94 % [2]:

- Narrow regular tachycardia → biphasic synchronized direct current shock 50–100 J
- Narrow irregular tachycardia → biphasic synchronized direct current shock 120–200 J
- Wide regular tachycardia → biphasic synchronized direct current shock 100 J
- Wide irregular tachycardia → biphasic NOT synchronized direct current shock 200 J

If there's no response to the first shock, it may be reasonable to increase the dose in a stepwise fashion.

Cardioversion with monophasic waveforms should begin at 200 J and increase in stepwise fashion if not successful [2].

In newborn, use $0.5 \to 2$ J/kg [3].

Heparin (low molecular weight or unfractionated heparin) should be administered before cardioversion in case of atrial flutter or atrial tachycardia and after it, depending on patients' features (CHA_2DS_2VASc – HAS BLED) [8].

In patients with implanted pacemaker or defibrillator pads, it should be positioned 8 cm from the device battery; anteroposterior paddle positioning and biphasic energy are recommended [2, 4, 8].

4.1.2 Patients in Stable Condition

The initial assessment should:

1. Distinguish between narrow and wide complex tachycardia.
2. Determine whether the rhythm is irregular or regular (<10 % of variation in cycle length).
3. Consider the rapidity of onset.
4. Identify sinus tachycardia (the theoretical upper rate is 220bpm minus the patient's age in years).

Supraventricular tachycardias have narrow QRS in 90 % of cases. Wide QRS complex could be due to pre-excitation through an accessory pathway or to bundle-branch block or to pacemaker stimulation. Previous ECG and ECG after termination of tachycardia can help to make the diagnosis.

While considering the patient's history, the clinician should assess the duration and frequency of episodes, the mode of onset, and possible triggers (including the intake of alcohol, caffeine or other drugs) as well as previous cardiac or other diseases or previous ECGs.

Supraventricular tachycardias have a sudden onset and termination, in contrast to sinus tachycardias or atrial tachycardias, which accelerate and decelerate gradually; however, some patients do not perceive the sudden onset of supraventricular tachycardia; furthermore, sometimes, they describe sudden onset and gradual offset due to reactive sinus tachycardia after termination of paroxysmal SVT. It may be misdiagnosed as panic disorder [5, 9].

Physical examination during episodes may reveal the "frog sign" which is a prominent jugular venous A waves due to atrial contraction against the closed tricuspid valve. After sinus rhythm is restored, physical examination is usually normal, but a careful examination is warranted to rule out evidence of structural heart disease [11, 12].

4.1.3 Management

4.1.3.1 Narrow QRS
If narrow QRS is present, atrioventricular conduction is certainly entirely through atrioventricular node. That's why maneuvers that increase vagal tone and block atrioventricular conduction are safe: they can interrupt tachycardias depending on AV node conduction (TRNAV or orthodromic TRAV) and can slow down those which don't depend on AV node conduction (atrial flutter or atrial fibrillation). They also interrupt focal tachycardia due to enhanced automaticity.

Physicians have these possibilities:

- *Vagal maneuvers* (Valsalva, carotid sinus massage, facial immersion in cold water, and bearing down). The efficacy is about 25 % [13]. Remember that carotid sinus massage is contraindicated in case of carotid stenosis.
- *Adenosine:* very short-acting endogenous nucleotide (<10 s). It blocks atrioventricular nodal conduction and terminates most of atrioventricular nodal reentrant tachycardias and atrioventricular reciprocating tachycardias as well as up to 80 % of atrial tachycardias [14–16]. Since it may also have proarrhythmic effect (atrial fibrillation in 12 % of patients), it must be administered under ECG monitoring with an accessible defibrillator.

  Common side effects include chest tightness, flushing, and a sense of dread. Avoid in asthmatic patients since it can produce bronchospasm; patients with autonomic failure and with cardiac transplant or patient chronically treated with antiarrhythmic drugs are more sensitive to adenosine [17]; that's why doses must be halved.

Way of administration and doses: 0.1–0.2 mg/kg (usually 6–12 mg) through peripheral vein; start with 6 mg in a rapid flush immediately followed by 20 ml of saline flush. If there is no effect, try again with 12 mg. Same dose for newborn.

- *Verapamil-diltiazem*: Intravenous verapamil and diltiazem are effective in interrupting tachycardias or can slow down AV conduction, but can cause hypotension thus are not recommended as first choice in the emergency setting [18]. They are contraindicated in heart failure and in newborn because of risk of cardiac arrest or atrioventricular dissociation [3, 19].
- *Electrical cardioversion*: best choice for atrial fibrillation and atrial flutter (typical o atypical) with onset within 48 h or in anticoagulated patients [8]. Biphasic synchronized shock ($50 \rightarrow 200$ J; $0.5 \rightarrow 2$ J/kg in infants) is recommended in sedated patient. Before cardioversion, a heparin bolus is recommended in all patients not yet anticoagulated. If there is no efficacy or there is arrhythmia recurrence, pharmacological therapy can be added.

Remember that:

- Sinus tachycardia is usually reactive to other causes so identification and treatment of them are required. No specific drug treatment is usually necessary.
- Atrial fibrillation and atrial flutter can give rise to endocardial thrombus which can cause stroke or thromboembolism: the risk is higher after 48 h of persistent tachycardia and in patients with some specific features ($CHA_2DS_2VASc > 1$). For this reason, anticoagulation (for at leat 3 weeks) is mandatory before cardioversion (or, in alternative, perform trans-esophageous echo to rule out intracardiac thrombi); in case of arrhythmias lasting more than 48 h or non-datable; nevertheless, heparin administration before cardioversion is preferable in all patients. For more details, see specific guidelines [16, 19–21].
- Patients with uncomplicated tachycardias and without cardiomyopathy can be discharged after sinus rhythm restoration; cardiological evaluation can be postponed.
- Sodium channel blockers increase both pacing threshold and the energy required to defibrillation [22, 23].
- Being genetic setting unknown, the effect of an antiarrhythmic drug given for the first time is *never* predictable. That's why administration of antiarrhythmic medications for the first time must be done under ECG monitoring lasting for at least the drug's half-time; after discharge, if chronic therapy is set up, ECG must be checked at the steady state (five half-times) (Fig. 4.2).

4.1.3.2 Wide QRS
Wide QRS can be due to preexisting or frequency-dependent bundle-branch block or to conduction over an accessory pathway. Nevertheless, the majority of wide QRS complex tachycardia has ventricular origin. If the patient is in stable hemodynamic condition, it is better to refer him/her to a specialist for diagnosis and treatment.

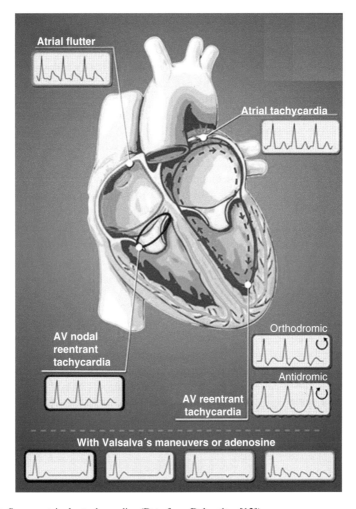

Fig. 4.2 Supraventricular tachycardias (Data from Delacrétaz [12])

4.2 What Cardiologists Should Know

Cardiologist should evaluate all patients with hemodynamic instability related to tachycardias after their stabilization with cardioversion in order to exclude or confirm the presence of cardiomyopathy, to decide the best medical treatment, and to decide for hospitalization or discharge and follow-up.

Non-urgent cardiological examination within few weeks can be reserved to uncomplicated tachycardias, in absence of cardiomyopathy, especially in case of preexisting diagnosis.

Cardiologist should know mechanisms underlying arrhythmias and modality of action of antiarrhythmic drugs in order to choose and combine them, to maximize efficacy and minimize proarrhythmic and side effects [22, 23], and to remove precipitating features as ischemia and electrolyte imbalance.

For this reason, the next part of the chapter is dedicated to pharmacology of antiarrhythmic drugs and basic electrophysiology.

At the end of the chapter, a scheme of therapies for each arrhythmia is provided.

4.2.1 Basic Electrophysiologic Principles

Every heart contraction is driven by inversion of cell potential from negative to positive. At the cell membrane site, this potential variation from negative to positive (depolarization) and back to negative (repolarization) is called action potential (AP). This is possible thanks to the activation in sequence of different channels driving ion currents (I) inward and outward the cell; every channel is designed to allow passage of its own specific ion and to do it only during a specific phase of AP (some channels open only at negative potential, other at positive). Potassium (K^+) is mainly inside the cell, while sodium (Na^+) is outside and calcium (Ca^{++}) is both outside and stored inside the cell; sodium and calcium are linked to one another. To generate cell depolarization, a specific potential threshold must be reached.

Action potential has been divided in five phases:

- 0 → Depolarization
- 1 → Fast repolarization
- 2 → Plateau
- 3 → Terminal repolarization
- 4 → Resting

During the first phase of action potential, cell membrane is depolarized, and no external stimulus can modify it (absolute refractoriness); during repolarization, external factors can excite the cell with "extra-AP" (relative refractoriness).

Propagation of action potential from a cell to another is called conduction and is characterized by a speed and a safety factor.

Action potential has different morphologies in different tissues (sinus node, AV node, atrioventricular cells). This is due to different kinds of channels and explains the heterogeneous effects of antiarrhythmic drugs on each cardiac tissue.

For example, AV node cell depolarization is mainly calcium mediated, while atrial and ventricular depolarization is sodium mediated; automaticity of sinus node is due to specific channels (HCN) which are permeable to both sodium and potassium and open only at very negative potentials (hyperpolarization).

Function alteration of ion channels (pathological, heart rate or drug mediated) or modifications of ion concentrations modify action potential in terms of duration, velocity of depolarization, or repolarization and determine abnormal rhythm propagation [5, 21].

4.2.2 Mechanisms of Arrhythmias

Arrhythmias are divided into focal and reentrant.

4.2.2.1 Focal

Focal supraventricular tachycardias are defined as an activation starting rhythmically from a small area in atria or AV junction and spreading out centrifugally. Focus can be single or multiple. Mechanism underlying focal tachycardias is automaticity, triggered activity, and micro-reentrant.

- *Triggered activity*: abnormal fluctuations of action potential occurring after or during the repolarization (phase 2–3 or 4 of action potential), which are able to depolarize cell membrane to the depolarization threshold; differently from automatic foci, they are linked to the previous action potential. Three kinds of triggered activities are known (Fig. 4.3):

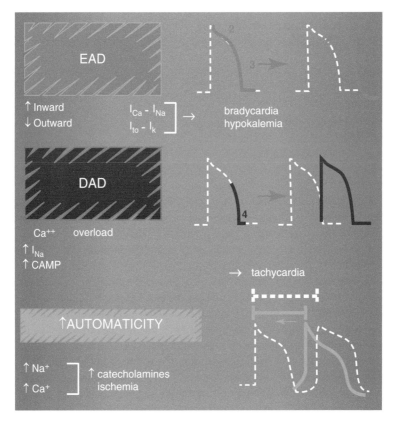

Fig. 4.3 Effects of early after depolarization (EAD), delayed after depolarization (DAD), and automaticity on action potential

(a) *Early after depolarization (EAD)* → occurring during repolarization (phases 2–3 of action potential), due to decreased potassium conductance (typically bradycardia, hypokalemia, or class III antiarrhythmic drugs). They are suppressed by factors that increase potassium outward current (*overdrive – tachycardias, K+ channels activators*) or suppress sodium/calcium inward currents (e.g., *magnesium*).

(b) *Delayed after depolarization (DAD)* → occurring during diastolic phase of action potential (phase 4) as consequence of Ca^{++} intracellular overload and Ca^{++} sparks due to increase of I_{Na} (ischemia or digoxin intoxication) or cAMP after beta-stimulation (tachycardia). They are suppressed by *beta-blockers, calcium channel blockers, vagal stimulation,* or *adenosine*.

(c) *Enhanced automaticity:* positive ionic influx (mostly inward calcium current) during phase 4 (diastolic) depolarization (normal automaticity is driven by sodium current while pathological by calcium). Beta-adrenergic stimulation enhances calcium current and facilitates these arrhythmias. Automatic tachycardias are the most common kind of focal arrhythmias and are characterized by sudden onset with a "warm-up" period. *Vagal stimulation, adenosine, beta-blockers,* or *calcium channel blockers* may suppress them.

Focal tachycardias are:

- *Atrial tachycardias* → P wave is generally visible with a morphology different from sinus one; 1:1 AV ratio is expected; heart rate can be very variable.
- *Inappropriate sinus tachycardia* → normal P wave morphology; 1:1 AV ratio; heart rate > 100 bpm not related to physiological needs.
- *Junctional tachycardia* → QRS not preceded by P; P wave can be visible after QRS, with morphology typical of AV junction origin (negative in DII–DIII and aVF, positive in V1 or not visible); similar to nodal or atrioventricular reentrant tachycardias; typical of infants.
- *Polymorphic atrial tachycardia/atrial fibrillation* → recurrent paroxysms of polymorphic premature beats starting with warm-up and degenerating in disorganized atrial activity; P wave is polymorphic and not always visible (during AF, sometime P is visible only in V1–V2 due to organization of atrial activity around tricuspid annulus).

4.2.2.2 Reentry

Reentry is a self-perpetuating circuit in which, during a single cardiac cycle, areas still depolarized and areas repolarized coexist. Reentry can be functional or anatomical. If the reentry circuit is >2–3 cm, it's classified as a macro-reentrant; if the reentry circuit is <2–3 cm, instead it's classified as micro (focal tachycardia) [25].

To have a reentry, the following features are required: unidirectional conduction (one way block usually due to extra beat), areas of different conduction rate (short and fast), and shortening of refractory period. Common triggers of reentry are sympathetic or parasympathetic stimulation, premature beats, and myocardial ischemia.

Wave length (WL) is the product of conduction velocity (CV) and refractory period (RP); WL is theoretical and is always shorter than the real one, so there is an excitable gap (EG) inside the circuit. Reentry has a wave front, a tail, and an excitable gap between them. Excitable gap is necessary to perpetuate reentry.

Factors eliminating the excitable gap block the reentrant circuit making the wave front crash on the tail. There are two ways to obtain it: to *increase the refractory period* (with potassium current blockers or sodium current blockers with slow kinetics) or to *increase the conduction velocity*. In addiction to drugs, the excitable gap can be suppressed stimulating the circuit at a rate just faster than the arrhythmia (overdrive pacing), possible in patients with dual chamber (or atrial) pacemakers.

Ablation can eliminate reentrant circuits by targeting areas of slow conduction that sustain circuit (called isthmus of the tachycardia) and blocking them (creating a permanent lesion with bidirectional block). When ablation lesion is incomplete, it can create an area of slower conduction that is potentially proarrhythmic.

Sometimes, the degree of increase of refractory period brought by drugs is not enough to interrupt tachycardia even at therapeutic concentration: this is more frequent in large anatomic circuit and with drugs that slow down propagation velocity as INa^+ blockers. In this situation arrhythmia became more stable and resistant to therapies. Examples are AVNRT slow/slow or permanent junctional reciprocating tachycardia (PJRT) after calcium or beta-blockers or transformation of atrial fibrillation (small circuit) in atrial flutter (large circuit) after flecainide or propafenone administration.

Reentrant tachycardias are:

- *Atrial flutter (typical and atypical)* → organized atrial rhythm; typical flutter is characterized by negative/positive sawtooth waves (F wave) in leads II, III, and aVF and positive in V_1; in atypical flutter, F waves have different axis depending on circuit; atrial heart rate is between 250 and 350 bpm (but can vary in patient previously treated with ablation or in patients taking antiarrhythmic drugs). In typical atrial flutter, circuit is counterclockwise around tricuspid annulus; slow conduction is between tricuspid annulus and inferior vena cava and conduction block along the crista terminalis and Eustachian ridge.
- *Post-incisional atrial tachycardia* → organized atrial activity due to reentrant around a scar; typical of patients with a history of cardiac surgery or catheter ablation.
- *AVNRT* → P wave arising from junction (negative in DII–DIII and aVF, positive in V1) with RP <PR; two limbs are slow and fast nodal pathways. Reentrant circuit is most of the time down through slow pathway and back through fast pathway (slow/fast), and P wave is visible as a pseudo-r′ in V1 or a pseudo-s′ in inferior leads (P can be not visible); in atypical AVNRT, circuit is down through slow or fast pathway and back through slow (slow/slow, fast/slow), and P wave is separated from QRS; RP >PR). The circuit is inside the AV node so that the

onset of atrioventricular block during tachycardia doesn't interrupt it (AVNRT can have 2:1 AV ratio).

- *AVRT*→reentrant circuit across AV node and accessory truck. It's called orthodromic when it passes from the atrium to the ventricle through AV node and back from the ventricle to the atrium through accessory pathway (RP >PR); it's called antidromic when anterograde wave front is through accessory pathway. The atria and ventricles are part of the circuit, and AV dissociation is not possible without interrupting tachycardia. Presence of pre-excitation is not diagnostic of AVRT (accessory pathway can be a "bystander" during AVNRT or atrial tachycardia, meaning that ventricles are partially or totally activated through the accessory pathway, which nevertheless is not part of the reentry circuit causing the arrhythmia). Evidence of tachycardia cycle length (=RR) augmentation of more than 35 ms (more and less 1 mm with 25 mm/s paper speed) in case of ipsilateral bundle brunch block is diagnostic of AVRT [24], because the ipsilateral block causes a lengthening of the circuit.

- *Permanent junctional reciprocating tachycardia (PJRT) – Mahaim tachycardia*→are rare AVRT through accessory pathway with particular features. PJRT is due to a septal accessory path with only retrograde conduction and decremental properties; it determines incessant narrow QRS tachycardia. Mahaim pathway is an accessory path with decremental properties generally right sided (from anterolateral atrial portion of tricuspid annulus to right ventricle or right bundle); in sinus rhythm, there is typically little or no pre-excitation; during antidromic tachycardia, the QRS is wide (150 ms), with left bundle block morphology, transition after V4.

4.2.3 Antiarrhythmic Drugs

Antiarrhythmic drugs are channel or receptor blockers. They bind specific sites on protein and modify its function with an affinity that varies on the ion channel state (open-inactivated-resting). Furthermore each drug has a specific rate of recovering from block which is a constant time ($T_{recovery}$).

This is why antiarrhythmic drugs that bind open channel, untie during resting state, and have long $T_{recovery}$ (as flecainide – 11 s) reach the steady state earlier having greater effect when a higher percentage of cells are depolarized as during ischemia or high heart rates (direct use dependence). Those drugs that, instead, own affinity for inactivated/resting channels (amiodarone or lidocaine) and own a very short $T_{recovery}$ (lidocaine – 0.1 s) have a greater effect (anti- and proarrhythmic!) under the condition that prolong action potential duration (as bradycardia-hypokalemia) and on rapidly driven tissue (ventricular tachycardia).

Antiarrhythmic drugs have been divided in four classes according to their main effect on action potential (Vaughan Williams classification) [25, 26]. However mostly all of them share properties among multiple classes (quinidine below to I°

class but have also III° class properties). Moreover, ivabradine, digoxin, and adenosine don't belong to any of the four classes (Table 4.1) (Fig. 4.4):

- INa+blockers (I class): shorten action potential, reduce propagation velocity, and act on refractoriness depending on kinetics (flecainide increase relative refractory period; lidocaine no); suppress EAD; reduce inotropism.
- Ica++ blockers (class IV): reduce propagation velocity; suppress abnormal automaticity, EAD, and DAD; reduce inotropism. All have direct use dependence.
- IK+ (class III): lengthening of action potential and of absolute refractory period. Increase inotropism. Have inverse use dependence. Proarrhythmic trough induction of EAD (during hypokalemia/bradycardia)

Key Messages
Remember that:
- *Electrolytes MUST be known, and their alterations MUST be correct before administering any antiarrhythmic drug!*
- Effect of antiarrhythmic drugs can be very different (and very dangerous) among patients with altered function of ion channels (channelopathies, myocardial ischemia) or variants of metabolic capacity or concomitant therapies [27–29]. Therefore, in patients with supraventricular arrhythmias and altered basal ECG (conduction disturbance, repolarization abnormalities), it is important to exclude those abnormalities and choose the correct therapy. When a channelopathy is suspected, further evaluation must be organized [30]; the decision about hospitalization or delayed ambulatory evaluation depends on the risk of arrhythmic death (arrhythmic instabilities, predisposing factors).
- Being genetic setting usually unknown, the *effect of an antiarrhythmic drug given for the first time is never predictable* [31]. That's why the first administration of any antiarrhythmic medications should be done under ECG monitoring lasting for at least the drug's half-time; after discharge, if chronic therapy is set up, ECG must be checked at steady state (five half-times).
- Ic are *effective on accessory pathway.*
- Ic are *poorly effective on atrial macro-reentrant tachycardias (flutter o postincisional)*; they slow atrial cycle length without interrupting tachycardia; if AV nodal conduction is enhanced (e.g., during exercise), they can promote 1:1 AV conduction. For this reason it's better to associate an AV blocker (Ca++ or Na+ blocker) to a Ic drug. Vernakalant is not effective on atrial flutter.
- Ic *have a marked negative inotropic effect*; if administered in rapid bolus, it causes broad hypotension even in people without cardiomyopathy so they must be administered under arterial pressure monitoring.
- *Calcium-blockers are dangerous in newborn* because of risk of cardiac arrest and are contraindicated in this setting [3, 19].
- *In newborn and children, beta-blockers are highly effective* especially if combined with amiodarone [32, 33]. Procainamide has also been demonstrated to be more effective than amiodarone in sinus rhythm conversion of pediatric SVT [34].

Table 4.1 The effects, doses, side effects, and contraindications of antiarrhythmic drugs

CLASS	DRUG		INTRAVENOUS	MAINTENANCE (day)	T 1/2	ELIMINATION	SIDE EFFECTS	CONTRAINDICATIONS
Ia → phase 0 conduction ↑ repolarization	DISOPYRAMIDE	↓ Na+,K+ ↑ M2	//	400-800 mg → 300/400 mg	4-8h	renal/hepatic	↑QT, TdP, gastrointestinal ailment, vasculitis, glaucoma, hypoglycemia	SA dysfuncion, bifascicular BBB, BAV II-III, severe heart failure, hypokalemia, CrCl <20 ml/min
	PROCAINAMIDE	↓ Na+,K+	30 mg/min (max 1 g) + 1-4 mg/min	250-1000 mg	3-4h	hepatic, renal	Hypotension, QRS widening, TdP	Severe heart failure, QRS widening > 50% basal
	QUINIDINA	↓ Na+,K+ ↑ M2,α,β		275mg(x3) 250-500mg (bid)		hepatic, renal	↑QT, diarrhea	
Ib → Na+ in phase 2 (effective on VT in abnormal tissue)	Lidocaine	↓ Na+	//	//	//		//	//
	Mexiletin	↓ Na+					//	//
	Tocainide	↓ Na+					//	//
	Phenytoin	↓ Na+					//	//
Ic → phase 0 conduction	FLECAINIDE	↓ Na+,K+ ↑ β	2 mg/Kg in 10'	3-5 mg/kg	12-20h	renal	Hypotension, negative inotropic effect, QRS widening, SA,AV block, dizziness, visual impairment, gastrointestinal ailment	Heart failure, Brugada Syndrome, LQT3, ischemic heart disease
	PRPPAFENONE	↓ Na+,β	2 mg/kg in 10'	10 mg/Kg	variable	hepatic		
	MORICIZINA	↓ Na+						
II β-blockers	ESMOLOL	↓ β	500 γ/Kg 1' → 20-200 γ/Kg/min	//	8'	esterases -	Bradicardia, Heart block, Hypotension, Negative inotropic effect, Bronchospasm	Asthma, II-III degree AV block, Heart failure
	METOPROLOL	↓ β1	5 mg in 2' → max 15 mg in 15'	50-200 mg	variable	hepatic		
	PROPANOLOL	↓ β1- β2	0,15-0,2 mg/Kg in 2'	80-240 mg	4 h	hepatic		
	ATENOLOL	↓ β1	2,5 mg in 1' → every 5', 25-100 mg	25-100 mg	6 h	renal		
	NADOLOL	↓ β1- β2	//	20-80 mg	20 h	renal		
	BISOPROLOL	↓ β1	//	2,5-10	//	hepatic/renal		
III ↑repolariziation	AMIODARON	↓ K+Na+, Ca++, β	5 mg/Kg in 20'-2h → 15 mg/Kg/24h	20 mg/Kg/week	240h	hepatic/renal	Skin discoloration, dyshyroidism, gastrointestinal up-set, hepatotoxicity, corneal deposits, tremor, optic neuropathy, pulmonary toxicity	LQT,hypokalemia Severe heart failure
	SOTALOL	↓ K+, β	//	3-5 mg/Kg (bid)	8 h	renal	↑QT, TdP, bradicardia, heart block, hypotension, negative inotropic effect, bronchospasm	LQT, hypokalemia, severe heart failure asthma, renal failure
	DOFETILIDE	↓ K+	//	1 mg	10h	renal/hepatic	↑QT, TdP (start in hospital)	LQT, ↓ K+, SA dysfuncion, AV II-III
	IBUTILIDE	↓ K+, ↑Na+	1 mg in 10'x2 (if <60Kg 0,01 mg/Kg)	//	2-12h	renal	↑QT, TdP, bradicardia	LQT, ↓ K,Mg++, SA dysfuncion, BAV II-III, recent MI
	DRONEDARON			800 mg		renal		LQT, -SA dysfuncion, BAV II-III, heart failure
	VERNAKALANT	↓ K+,Na+	//	//	//	//	//	
IV Ca++ Antagonist	VERAPAMIL	↓ Ca++	5mg/Kgin5' → max10mg	120-480 mg	3-7 h	hepatic	Bradicardia, SA,AV block, hypotension, negative inotropic effect	II-III degree AV block, heart failure, newborn
	DILTIAZEM	↓ Ca++	0,25-0,35 mg/Kg in 2' → 5-15 mg/h	180-360 mg	4h	hepatic		
	ADENOOSINE	↓ A1	0,1-0,2 mg/Kg	//	<10''	esterases	bronchospasm, flushing	asthma
	DIGOXIN	↓ M2	1 mg/12-24 h	0,125-0,375 mg	36h	renal	tachyarrhythmias, SA,AV block	hypokalemia, severe renal disease
	IVABRADINE	↑↓	//	2,5-7,5 mg (bid)	12 h	renal	bradicardia, bradicardia-mediated VT and AF, phosphenes, headache	bradyarrhythmias, LQT, severe heart failure

Different colors identify the four classes of Vaughan Williams classification; in *black* drugs not belonging to any class. Drugs without indications for supraventricular tachycardias are only mentioned

Fig. 4.4 Major effects of antiarrhythmic drugs on action potential

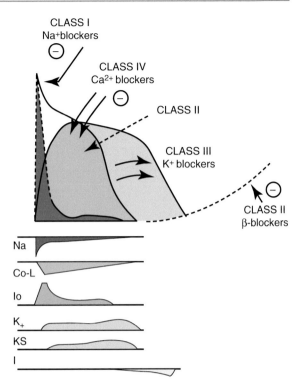

- *Newborn and children aren't* "small adults": they have different metabolism that MUST be known (usually they are better metabolizer than old people); drug's doses must be setup on body weight.
- Amiodarone is effective on different substrates due to its multiple antiarrhythmic affect (class from I to IV).
- *Risk of EAD due to a drug that blocks IK is reduced by addition of a INa/ICa blocker* (as quinidine + verapamil).
- *Supraventricular tachycardias can be associated with troponin level and/or ST abnormalities that rise in absence of coronary artery disease* [35, 36]. Suspicion of coronary syndrome must be based on risk factors, symptoms, ECG, or echocardiographic alteration.
- *Catheter ablation is safe and highly effective in curing supraventricular arrhythmias permanently*. It is a reasonable option of antiarrhythmic therapies in most of tachycardias and must be considered and proposed to patients [4, 37, 38] (Fig. 4.5).

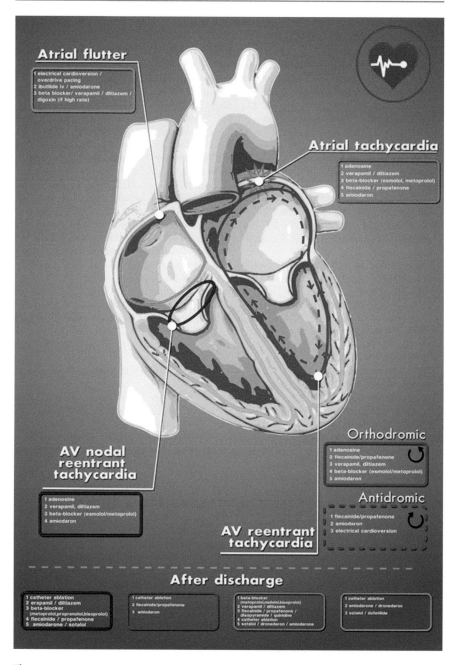

Fig. 4.5 Mechanisms, acute and long-term treatment of major supraventricular arrhythmias due to reentry circuits

References

1. Orejarena LA, Vidaillet Jr H, DeStefano F, et al. Paroxysmal supraventricular tachycardia in the general population. J Am Coll Cardiol. 1998;31:150–7.
2. Neumar RW, Otto CW, Link MS, et al. Part 8: adult advanced cardiovascular life support: 2010 American Heart Association Guidelines for Cardiopulmonary Resuscitation and Emergency Cardiovascular Care. Circulation. 2010;122 Suppl 3:S729–67.
3. Kleinman ME, Chameides L, Schexnayder SM, Samson RA, Hazinski MF, Atkins DL, Berg MD, de Caen AR, Fink EL, Freid EB, Hickey RW, Marino BS, Nadkarni VM, Proctor LT, Qureshi FA, Sartorelli K, Topjian A, van der Jagt EW, Zaritsky AL. Part 14: pediatric advanced life support: 2010 American Heart Association Guidelines for Cardiopulmonary Resuscitation and Emergency Cardiovascular Care. Circulation. 2010;122(18 Suppl 3):S876–908.
4. Blomström-Lundqvist C, Scheinman MM, Aliot EM, Alpert JS, Calkins H, Camm AJ, Campbell WB, Haines DE, Kuck KH, Lerman BB, Miller DD, Shaeffer CW, Stevenson WG, Tomaselli GF, Antman EM, Smith Jr SC, Alpert JS, Faxon DP, Fuster V, Gibbons RJ, Gregoratos G, Hiratzka LF, Hunt SA, Jacobs AK, Russell Jr RO, Priori SG, Blanc JJ, Budaj A, Burgos EF, Cowie M, Deckers JW, Garcia MA, Klein WW, Lekakis J, Lindahl B, Mazzotta G, Morais JC, Oto A, Smiseth O, Trappe HJ, European Society of Cardiology Committee, NASPE-Heart Rhythm Society. ACC/AHA/ESC guidelines for the management of patients with supraventricular arrhythmias – executive summary. a report of the American college of cardiology/American heart association task force on practice guidelines and the European society of cardiology committee for practice guidelines (writing committee to develop guidelines for the management of patients with supraventricular arrhythmias) developed in collaboration with NASPE-Heart Rhythm Society. J Am Coll Cardiol. 2003;42(8):1493–531.
5. Bonow R, Mann D, Zipes D, Libby P. Braunwald's heart disease. 9th ed. Philadelphia: Elsevier Inc; 2012.
6. Rijnbeek PR, Witsenburg M, Schrama E, Hess J, Kors JA. New normal limits for the paediatric electrocardiogram. Eur Heart J. 2001;22(8):702–11.
7. Schwartz PJ, Garson Jr A, Paul T, Stramba-Badiale M, Vetter VL, Villain E, Wren C. Linee guida Linee guida per l'interpretazione dell'elettrocardiogramma neonatale Task Force della Società Europea di Cardiologia. Ital Heart J Suppl. 2003;4(2):138–53.
8. Dankner R, Shahar A, Novikov I, Agmon U, Ziv A, Hod H. Treatment of stable atrial fibrillation in the emergency department: a population-based comparison of electrical direct-current versus pharmacological cardioversion or conservative management. Cardiology. 2009;112(4):270–8.
9. Lessmeier TJ, Gamperling D, Johnson Liddon V, et al. Unrecognized paroxysmal supraventricular tachycardia: potential for misdiagnosis as panic disorder. Arch Intern Med. 1997;157:537–43.
10. Brunton L, Blumenthal D, Buxton I, Parker K. Goodman and Gilman's. Manual of pharmacology and therapetutics. New York: McGraw-Hill Companies; 2008.
11. Link MS. Clinical practice. Evaluation and initial treatment of supraventricular tachycardia. N Engl J Med. 2012;367(15):1438–48.
12. Delacrétaz E. Supraventricular tachycardia. N Engl J Med. 2006;354(10):1039–51.
13. Lim SH, Anantharaman V, Teo WS, Goh PP, Tan AT. Comparison of treatment of supraventricular tachycardia by Valsalva maneuver and carotid sinus massage. Ann Emerg Med. 1998;31:30–5.
14. diMarco JP, Sellers TD, Lerman BB, Greenberg ML, Berne RM, Belardinelli L. Diagnostic and therapeutic use of adenosine in patients with supraventricular tachyarrhythmias. J Am Coll Cardiol. 1985;6:417–25.
15. Paul T, Pfammatter JP. Adenosine: an effective and safe antiarrhythmic drug in pediatrics. Pediatr Cardiol. 1997;18(2):118–26.
16. January CT, Wann LS, Alpert JS, Calkins H, Cigarroa JE, Cleveland Jr JC, Conti JB, Ellinor PT, Ezekowitz MD, Field ME, Murray KT, Sacco RL, Stevenson WG, Tchou PJ, Tracy CM, Yancy CW. 2014 AHA/ACC/HRS guideline for the management of patients with atrial fibrillation: a report of the American College of Cardiology/American Heart Association Task Force on Practice Guidelines and the Heart Rhythm Society. Circulation. 2014;130(23):e199–267.

17. Biaggioni I, Olafsson B, Robertson RM, Hollister AS, Robertson D. Cardiovascular and respiratory effects of adenosine in conscious man: evidence for chemoreceptor activation. Circ Res. 1987;61:779–86.
18. Delaney B, Loy J, Kelly AM. The relative efficacy of adenosine versus verapamil for the treatment of stable paroxysmal supraventricular tachycardia in adults: a meta-analysis. Eur J Emerg Med. 2011;18:148–52.
19. Roguin N, Shapir Y, Blazer S, Zeltzer M, Berant M. The use of calcium gluconate prior to verapamil in infants with paroxysmal supraventricular tachycardia. Clin Cardiol. 1984; 7(11):613–6.
20. Camm AJ, Kirchhof P, Lip GY, Schotten U, Savelieva I, Ernst S, Van Gelder IC, Al-Attar N, Hindricks G, Prendergast B, Heidbuchel H, Alfieri O, Angelini A, Atar D, Colonna P, De Caterina R, De Sutter J, Goette A, Gorenek B, Heldal M, Hohloser SH, Kolh P, Le Heuzey JY, Ponikowski P, Rutten FH. Guidelines for the management of atrial fibrillation: the Task Force for the Management of Atrial Fibrillation of the European Society of Cardiology (ESC). European Heart Rhythm Association; European Association for Cardio-Thoracic Surgery. Eur Heart J. 2010;31(19):2369–429.
21. Camm AJ, Lip GY, De Caterina R, Savelieva I, Atar D, Hohnloser SH, Hindricks G, Kirchhof P, ESC Committee for Practice Guidelines (CPG). 2012 focused update of the ESC Guidelines for the management of atrial fibrillation: an update of the 2010 ESC Guidelines for the management of atrial fibrillation. Developed with the special contribution of the European Heart Rhythm Association. Eur Heart J. 2012;33:2719–47.
22. Brunton L, Blumenthal D, Buxton I, Parker K. Goodman and Gilman's. Manual of pharmacology and therapeutics. New York: McGraw-Hill Companies; 2008.
23. Opie LH, Gersh BJ. Drug for the heart. 7th edn. Philadelphia: Saunders Elsevier; 2009.
24. Yang Y, Cheng J, Glatter K, Dorostkar P, Modin GW, Scheinman MM. Quantitative effects of functional bundle branch block in patients with atrioventricular reentranttachycardia. Am J Cardiol. 2000;85(7):826–31.
25. Vaughan Williams EM. Classification of antidysrhythmic drugs. Pharmacol Ther B. 1975;1:115–38.
26. Members of the Sicilian Gambit. The search for novel antiarrhythmic strategies. Sicilian Gambit. Eur Heart J. 1998;19:1178–96.
27. Antzelevitch C, Brugada P, Borggrefe M, Brugada J, Ramon B, Domenico C, Ihor G, Herve LM, Koonlawee N, Andres Ricardo Perez R, Wataru S, Eric S-B, Hanno T, Arthur W. Brugada syndrome: report of the second consensus conference: endorsed by the Heart Rhythm Society and the European Heart Rhythm Association. Circulation. 2005;111:659–70.
28. Antzelevitch C. J wave syndromes: molecular and cellular mechanisms. J Electrocardiol. 2013;46(6):510–8.
29. Minoura Y, Di Diego JM, Barajas-Martinez H, Zygmunt AC, Hu D, Sicouri S, Antzelevitch C. Ionic and cellular mechanisms underlying the development of acquired Brugada syndrome in patients treated with antidepressants. J Cardiovasc Electrophysiol. 2012;23(4):423–32.
30. Ackerman MJ, Priori SG, Willems S, Berul C, Brugada R, Calkins H, Camm AJ, Ellinor PT, Gollob M, Hamilton R, Hershberger RE, Judge DP, Le Marec H, McKenna WJ, Schulze-Bahr E, Semsarian C, Towbin JA, Watkins H, Wilde A, Wolpert C, Zipes DP, Heart Rhythm Society (HRS); European Heart Rhythm Association (EHRA). HRS/EHRA expert consensus statement on the state of genetic testing for the channelopathies and cardiomyopathies: this document was developed as a partnership between the Heart Rhythm Society (HRS) and the European Heart Rhythm Association (EHRA). Europace. 2011;13(8):1077–109.
31. Van Opstal JM, Volders PG, Crijns HJ. Provocation of silence. Europace. 2009;11(3):385–7.
32. Drago F, Mazza A, Guccione P, Mafrici A, Di Liso G, Ragonese P. Amiodarone used alone or in combination with propranolol: a very effective therapy for tachyarrhythmias in infants and children. Pediatr Cardiol. 1998;19(6):445–9.
33. Akin A, Karagöz T, Aykan HH, Özer S, Alehan D, Özkutlu S. The efficacy of amiodarone-propranolol combination for the management of childhood arrhythmias. Pacing Clin Electrophysiol. 2013;36(6):727–31.

34. Chang PM, Silka MJ, Moromisato DY, Bar-Cohen Y. Amiodarone versus procainamide for the acute treatment of recurrent supraventricular tachycardia in pediatric patients. Circ Arrhythm Electrophysiol. 2010;3(2):134–40.
35. Zellweger MJ, Schaer BA, Cron TA, Pfisterer ME, Osswald S. Elevated troponin levels in absence of coronary artery disease after supraventricular tachycardia. Swiss Med Wkly. 2003;133:439–41.
36. Redfearna DP, Ratibb K, Marshalla HJ, Griffitha MJ. Supraventricular tachycardia promotes release of troponin I in patients with normal coronary arteries. Int J Cardiol. 2005;102:521–2.
37. Macías Gallego A, Díaz-Infante E, García-Bolao I. Spanish catheter ablation registry. 10th official report of the Spanish Society of Cardiology Working Group on Electrophysiology and Arrhythmias (2010). Rev Esp Cardiol. 2011;64(12):1147–53.
38. Scheinman M, Calkins H, Gillette P, Klein R, Lerman BB, Morady F, Saksena S, Waldo A, North American Society of Pacing and Electrophysiology. NASPE policy statement on catheter ablation: personnel, policy, procedures, and therapeutic recommendations. Pacing Clin Electrophysiol. 2003;26(3):789–99.

Atrial Flutter and Fibrillation in the Emergency Setting

5

Ermanno Dametto, Martino Cinquetti,
Federica Del Bianco, and Matteo Cassin

5.1 Focus on the Topic

Atrial fibrillation (AF) is a supraventricular arrhythmia characterised by uncoordinated atrial activation which determines on the electrocardiogram (ECG) the presence of fibrillatory waves of different timing, shape and amplitude, associated with an irregular and frequently rapid ventricular response (Fig. 5.1). It is the most frequent arrhythmia with a prevalence of 1.5–2 % in the general population [1], increasing with age and is the most frequent cause of arrhythmic access to the emergency department (ED), 1.5 % in "FIRE" and 3.1 % in "HERMES-AF" registries [2, 3] and hospitalisation (3.3 % in "FIRE" registry [2]).

European (ESC 2010) [4] and US (AHA/ACC/HRS 2014) [5] guidelines (GL) classify AF as *first diagnosed* or *recurrent*. Recurrent AF episodes are defined as *paroxysmal* if they terminate spontaneously (AHA/ACC/HRS 2014 GL [5] include also AF treated with cardioversion within 7 days), *persistent* (lasting longer than 7 days), *long-lasting persistent* (continuous for more than 12 months with intention of rhythm control strategy) or *permanent* (further attempts to restore and/or maintain sinus rhythm excluded).

AF may be asymptomatic, so the patient may be referred to the ED by a general physician for an occasional finding of irregular heart rhythm, or symptomatic. Symptoms described on arrival at the ED are most frequently palpitations (69.2 %), followed by dyspnoea (27.5 %), congestive heart failure (10.9 %), fatigue (105), angina (9 %), pulmonary oedema (4.5 %), syncope (3.3 %), transitory ischaemic attack (TIA) or stroke (2.2 %) [2]. Apart from acute symptoms, atrial fibrillation

E. Dametto (✉) • F. Del Bianco, • M. Cassin
Cardiology Unit, Presidio Ospedaliero di Pordenone, AAS5-Azienda per l'Assistenza Sanitaria n.5 "Friuli Occidentale", Pordenone, Italy
e-mail: ermanno.dametto@gmail.com

M. Cinquetti
Cardiovascular Department, Ospedali Riuniti and University of Trieste, Trieste, Italy

© Springer International Publishing Switzerland 2016
M. Zecchin, G. Sinagra (eds.), *The Arrhythmic Patient in the Emergency Department: A Practical Guide for Cardiologists and Emergency Physicians*, DOI 10.1007/978-3-319-24328-3_5

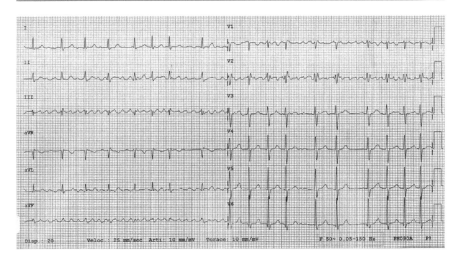

Fig. 5.1 *Atrial fibrillation* with moderately fast ventricular response (about 100 bpm). RR intervals are irregular and coarse F waves are visible

causes a fivefold risk of stroke, a threefold risk of heart failure and doubles dementia and mortality [5]. Furthermore, it reduces the quality of life [6]. For stroke, risk stratification and treatment of *nonvalvular* and *valvular AF* are distinguished. Valvular AF carries a very high thromboembolic risk if not anticoagulated: in patients with mitral stenosis and AF it is about 20 times over patients not affected by AF. Definition of valvular AF is not univocal; according to the AHA/ACC/HRS 2014 Guidelines, it is defined as AF associated with rheumatic mitral stenosis, a mechanical or bioprosthetic heart valve or mitral valve repair [5].

Atrial flutter (AFL) is less common (about 10 % of ED admissions for AF or AFL were due to AFL in the "FIRE" registry [2]) but shares similar clinical features and treatment with AF. It is a macroreentrant atrial arrhythmia with regular atrial activation and shows electrocardiographically continuous atrial activity in at least one lead which may have various morphologies depending on the location of the circuit. The ventricular rate is usually regular due to a fixed atrioventricular (AV) conduction rate, mostly 2:1 with a frequency of 120–150 bpm (Fig. 5.2), but may be slower or irregular due to a variable AV conduction rate.

Both arrhythmias are usually associated with cardiovascular pathologies, mostly hypertension (64 %) but also coronary artery disease (32 %), heart failure (32 %), valvular hear disease (26 %) and cardiomyopathy (10 %). Chronic obstructive pulmonary disease (COPD) may be associated in 13 % of the patients and thyroid disease in 9 %. In about 10 %, none of these comorbidities are found, and the arrhythmia is called "lone atrial fibrillation" (or flutter), if the patient is younger than 65 years old [7].

Acute diseases may be associated with AF/AFL like myocardial infarction, pulmonary embolism, pneumonia, severe infections, alcohol abuse, drug toxicity, hypothermia and electrolyte abnormalities [8].

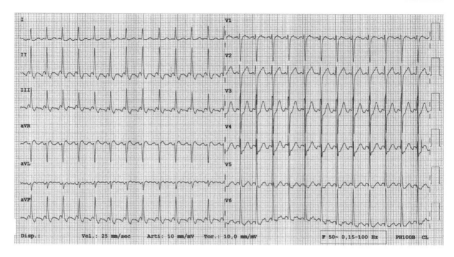

Fig. 5.2 *Atrial flutter with 2:1 AV conduction and quite rapid ventricular rate* of 150 bpm. Regular RR intervals

5.2   What Physicians Working in ED Should Know

The ED physician has several tasks:

1. *Rule out severe clinical instability*

Altered mental status, hypotension, pulmonary oedema and ongoing ischemia necessitate acute electrical cardioversion (ECV) once diagnosis of AF/AFL is confirmed and is thought to be the primary cause [9], at least if there is no prompt response to rate control therapy [4, 5, 10].

2. *Diagnosis of the arrhythmia*

The pulse presents irregular in case of AF but is usually regular in case of flutter. Electrocardiographic diagnosis of AF is usually easy for the irregular RR intervals and f waves. Atrial flutter appears usually as a regular arrhythmia due to fixed conduction rate, mostly 2:1 with ventricular rates around 120–150 bpm, but may be less or conduction may be variable. When rapid conduction is present, the flutter waves may not be so evident. In these cases and if the patient is stable, we recommend to perform a continuous 12-lead ECG registration during carotid sinus massage (after exclusion of any carotid bruit) or adenosine infusion (6, 12 or 18 mg bolus followed by 20 ml saline solution flush) to clear up differential diagnosis with other supraventricular arrhythmias and to record the flutter wave morphology, which helps the cardiologist to define the long-term therapeutic approach (e.g. radiofrequency ablation). *Typical atrial flutter* (also called *cavotricuspid isthmus-dependent atrial flutter*) is a macroreentrant circuit posterior to the tricuspid annulus, crossing the

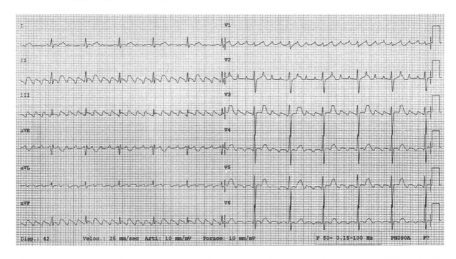

Fig. 5.3 *Typical atrial flutter with counterclockwise atrial activation (common atrial flutter)* with 4:1 AV conduction, 70 bpm. Atrial flutter waves are clearly seen: negative in inferior leads and positive in V1

isthmus between the inferior vena cava orifice and tricuspid annulus. Activation sequence is more frequently counterclockwise (downwards the right atrial free wall and upwards the interatrial septum), and in this case, the arrhythmia is called *common atrial flutter* or *counterclockwise AFL* (Fig. 5.3). Less common is *clockwise typical atrial flutter*, also called *reverse AFL* (Fig. 5.4). On ECG, the former shows classical "sawtooth" flutter waves with negative polarity in inferior leads and positive in V1, and the latter shows flutter waves with positive polarity in the inferior leads and negative in V1. Atypical flutters (noncavotricuspid isthmus dependent) show flutter waves with other morphologies (Fig. 5.5) [5].

In patients with AFL treated with flecainide or propafenone sometimes rapid 1:1 AV conduction is favoured due to flutter wave slowing. This phenomenon is frequently accompained by conduction aberrancy and QRS widening (Fig. 5.6).

In patients with Wolff–Parkinson–White Syndrome, a *pre-excited AF* (Fig. 5.7) is characterised by irregular RR intervals with various degrees of QRS widening (various degrees of fusion between accessory pathway and nodal conduction). In case of fast conduction properties of the accessory pathway, ventricular rate can be extremely high, possibly leading to severe haemodynamic consequences or even to ventricular fibrillation. *Pre-excited AFL* appears as a wide QRS tachycardia.

3. *Clinical history and physical examination for evaluation of concomitant heart disease and comorbidities*

A complete medical history including previous cardiac and noncardiac diseases, history of former AF, medication use and drug or alcohol abuse should be obtained. Onset of the current AF episode should be carefully defined as it is a crucial point for decision making, in particular, it has to be cleared if onset is within or more than

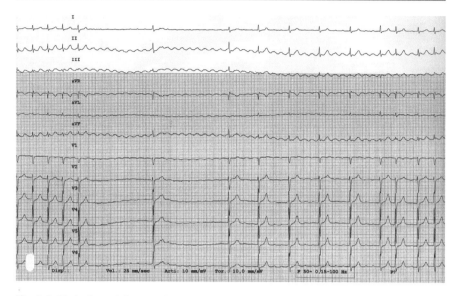

Fig. 5.4 *Typical atrial flutter with clockwise atrial activation (reverse atrial flutter) during adenosine injection.* Initially 2:1 AV conduction, 150 bpm and masked flutter waves. A marked conduction slowing follows, unmasking flutter waves: positive in inferior leads and negative in V1. Diagnosis was confirmed by electrophysiological study

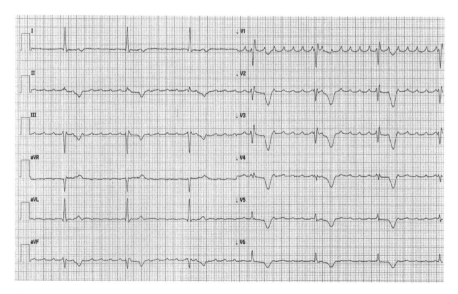

Fig. 5.5 *Atypical atrial flutter:* flutter waves are positive in inferior leads and in V1

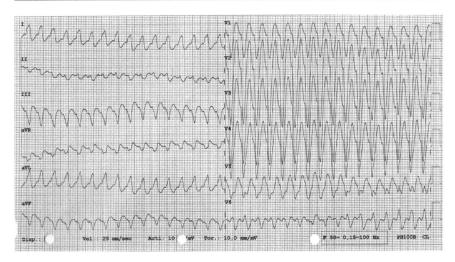

Fig. 5.6 *Atrial flutter with 1:1 AV conduction and aberrancy* 190 bpm (during i.v. flecainide infusion). Flutter waves are not visible. Resembles a wide QRS tachycardia

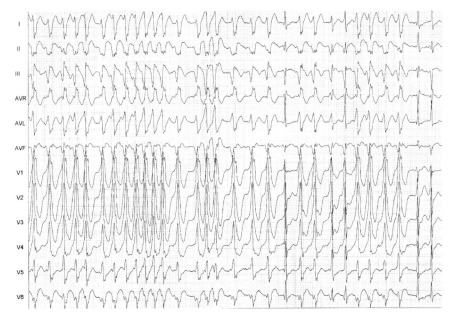

Fig. 5.7 *Pre-excited atrial fibrillation with fast AV conduction*, at times near 300 bpm. Bizarre wide QRS morphology with irregular RR intervals. In between, there are a few beats with normal QRS, conducted through the AV node

48 h (time within acute cardioversion without previous anticoagulation can be considered). Frequently, AF presents as continuous palpitations with acute onset. In this case, onset definition is easy. Other times, palpitations are perceived intermittently

or other symptoms dominate as dyspnoea or fatigue which can be vague. In these cases, it can be of help if patients are used to evaluate daily their pulse (often evaluated together with arterial pressure in the hypertensive). If onset of AF cannot be clearly dated, the arrhythmia should be regarded as "AF of undefined onset".

Physical examination should initially be aimed to vital signs like blood pressure, pulse frequency, signs of pulmonary or peripheral congestion and oxygen saturation. Cardiac assessment should include evaluation of heart sounds and murmurs and a careful evaluation of both arterial and jugular pulse (to assess the rhythm and possible AV dissociation).

Laboratory tests should be tailored to patient's presentation. A complete blood count, serum electrolytes, renal and hepatic function tests, coagulation status and thyroid-stimulating hormone should be routinely obtained. Brain natriuretic peptide, troponin I or T, C-reactive protein and D-dimer test help ruling out heart failure, myocardial ischemia, concomitant inflammatory or infectious disease and pulmonary embolism if these conditions are suspected.

Thyroid disease is not uncommon in AF patients and overt hyperthyroidism is associated in about 4 % of AF patients [11]. Thyroid-stimulating hormone is a reliable screening tool which can be applied in some EDs and may help in decision making (choosing rate control strategy or defining contraindication for amiodarone use [12].

An urgent echocardiogram should be performed in haemodynamically compromised patients [4]. Alternatively, a focused ultrasonography performed by the ED physician can determine underlying cardiac condition like structural heart disease, pericardial effusion and pulmonary embolism, or clarify causes of shock or hypotension and guide resuscitation by volume repletion measuring the inferior vena cava diameter. Ultrasound competence is not uniformly available among ED physicians, but a focused examination of the heart may help guiding therapy in AF management [13]. However, a complete echocardiographic examination should be performed as part of initial evaluation [4, 5, 14] as soon as possible, even on outpatient basis in stable patients.

4. *Symptom relief by cardioversion (electrical or pharmacological) or rate control*

Unstable patients   In patients with haemodynamic compromise like hypotension, pulmonary oedema or ongoing myocardial ischemia thought to result mainly from acute AF or AFL, electrical cardioversion is indicated [9], especially if it does not respond promptly to pharmacological rate control measures [4, 5, 10].

Anticoagulation with low molecular weight heparin (LMWH) or unfractionated heparin (UFH) should be initiated as soon as possible. Do not delay ECV if the patient is extremely unstable [9]. In the author's opinion if the patient is hypotensive, ECV is preferable, whereas if pulmonary oedema or myocardial ischaemia is present, rate control should be tried first.

Atrial fibrillation can be an epiphenomenon of an "alternative" primary diagnosis, and in these cases, mortality rate is high (11 % in the study of Atzema et al. [15]). Patients may present with vague symptoms. Scheuermeyer et al. [16] reported on a series of patients with underlying medical illness like sepsis, acute coronary syndrome (ACS), decompensated heart failure, pulmonary embolism, obstructive pulmonary disease exacerbation, acute renal failure and gastrointestinal bleedings. Those who underwent immediate rate or rhythm control attempts suffered a much higher complication rate (40.7 %) than those who did not (7.1 %) and were unlikely to achieve success. So it is more advisable to delay rhythm management strategies and manage these patients first correcting the primary acute disease, administrating intravenous fluids guided by bedside echocardiography (to assess volume status) and performing frequent reassessments while waiting for confirmatory diagnostic tests [16].

Stable patients with recent-onset AF (<48 h) There is still controversy on optimal management of these patients, being rate and rhythm control the two alternative strategies without clear-cut evidence favouring one or the other. *Rate control strategy* in the ED consists of pharmacological control of ventricular rate and anticoagulation treatment if indicated. With *rhythm control strategy*, the patient is cardioverted to sinus rhythm (SR) either pharmacologically or electrically, usually discharged from the ED and followed as outpatient afterwards. A delayed cardioversion (CV) after at least 3 weeks of adequate anticoagulation can be planned in some patients if the initial rate control strategy is not well tolerated.

Although several trials on AF patients like the AFFIRM [17] did not find significant differences on the main clinical outcomes between rate and rhythm control, the latter seems the preferred strategy worldwide in the long treatment of AF [18, 19]. General indications for preference of either strategy are listed in Italian guidelines on AF management [20]: rhythm control strategy should be the option for (1) patients with first AF episode (taking into account also age and comorbidities) and (2) for patients with recurrent AF with high probability of long-term sinus rhythm maintenance, or in whom rate control proved uneffective or if AF determines negative haemodynamic effects. Rate control strategy is preferred for (1) patients refractory to antiarrhythmic therapy, with frequent AF relapses non-candidable to AF ablation or not candidable to rhythm control strategy because of age or underlying heart disease and (2) for older asymptomatic patients with persistent AF or older patients with recurrent AF, heart failure and poor ventricular function.

As far as ED practice concerns, there is a considerable variability among different countries: rate control strategy is largely favoured in the USA (74 %), while in Canada, most patients undergo cardioversion (66 %). The UK and Australia adopt rate or rhythm control in equal proportions [21].

In our clinic, rhythm control is generally the preferred management strategy.

The theoretical advantages of an aggressive rhythm control approach are rapid discharge without hospital admission, immediate resumption of normal activities, potential avoidance of medications and minimization of healthcare resources and costs. In addition, with rate control strategy, many patients can derive physical and psychological inconvenience maintaining the arrhythmia and drugs after discharge [22].

A recent review of five studies involving 1593 cases undergoing ED cardioversion [23] demonstrated that success rate was high (around 90 %), with a discharge rate of about 90 % and a complication rate generally lower than 5 %, exceptionally leading to hospital admission. Thromboembolic complication rate was very low (0.06 %). So in selected patients with recent-onset AF, ED physicians should feel comfortable with this approach which should ideally be standardised by a local ED protocol and include timely and appropriate follow-up. The first description of an ED protocol dealing with recent-onset AF or flutter was the "Ottawa Aggressive Protocol" [24]. Excluding patients presenting with AF onset >48 h or of unknown duration and those with other primary diagnosis necessitating admission, it involved sequential pharmacologic and, when indicated, electrical cardioversion by the emergency physician. It allowed discharge of 96.8 % of the 660 enrolled patients, 93.3 % of those in sinus rhythm, after a median length of stay of 4.9 h overall. Adverse outcomes, mainly transient hypotension, occurred in 7.6 % and only 3.2 % of patients required hospitalisation. No patient died or suffered a stroke. Despite these encouraging results, limited data help guide emergency physicians on which AF patients can be safely managed as outpatients (see below). An interesting implementation of an ED cardioversion protocol for acute AF patients after exclusion of high-risk features was described by Bellone et al. [13]; their workup included morphological echocardiographic investigation before treatment by certified emergency physicians, which has the potential of improving the risk stratification and the therapeutical choice.

Another management strategy consists in conservative "wait-and-watch approach" which relies on the known discrete likelihood of spontaneous cardioversion of recent-onset AF (from 20 % up to 68 % in the study of Danias et al. [25]); early (<24 h) presentation is the best predictor of spontaneous cardioversion. Patients may be discharged on rate control medication and anticoagulation if appropriate and scheduled for return visit to ED to permit CV within the 48 h period [26] from symptom onset if AF persists, or may be admitted to an ED observation unit, reassessed after some hours and eventually cardioverted if AF persists [27]. This strategy can be applied following the patient's preference but may be an option if ED is overcrowded.

Stable patients with AF onset >48 h or with AF of uncertain onset If the patient has properly been anticoagulated for at least the preceeding 3 weeks, acute cardioversion can be considered as an alternative to rate control. On the contrary, in nonanticoagulated patients, rate control is generally the most appropriate strategy. In the acute setting, the target ventricular rate should usually be 80–100 bpm [4]. Once rhythm control is achieved and anticoagulation started, the patient can be considered for discharge and referred to a cardiologist or a general practitioner. If adequate rate control is not achieved, the patient is still symptomatic or if new ventricular dysfunction is to be detected, cardioversion should be considered: the patient must be fully anticoagulated independently of the thromboembolic risk (start with UFH or LMWH for immediate action and bridge then with vitamin K antagonists; novel anticoagulants may be used as alternative), then undergo a transoesophageal echocardiogram (TEE) to exclude intracardiac thrombi and finally electrically cardioverted. Anticoagulation should be continued at least 4 weeks or indefinitely, according on the thromboembolic risk profile. If thrombosis is detected, the patient should undergo another TEE after at least 3 weeks of effective anticoagulation and if it has resolved undergo ECV thereafter [4, 5, 10].

According to the Canadian Guidelines 2014 [10], the TEE-based CV approach should also be applied for a AF patients presenting <48 h after AF onset if high-risk features like valvular AF or stroke/TIA in the last 6 months are present.

5. *Antithrombotic therapy*

It is generally believed that antithrombotic therapy is the mainstay of AF management in any care setting, as from this therapy, most of prognostic benefit in terms of morbidity (stroke prevention) and mortality has to be gained. Nevertheless, it is still much underprescribed, usually in less than 55 % of AF patients, as results from studies are conducted in different settings. EDs constitute excellent opportunities to start thromboprophylaxis in the absence of contraindications and help filling this gap [3]. Treatment options include LMWH or UFH, vitamin K antagonists (VKAs) and novel oral anticoagulants (NOACs).

Immediate anticoagulation can be obtained with unfractionated heparin (i.v. bolus of 80 UI/kg followed by continuous i.v. infusion adjusted to an activated partial thromboplastin time of twice the control value (initially 18 UI/kg/h)) [28] or LMWH (most popular being enoxaparin 100 UI/kg BID) based on ACUTE II [29] ad ACE trials [30]. Heparin therapy is generally used as bridging with VKAs which have a delayed onset of action which takes some days.

At present, three NOACs have been tested for AF cardioversion (prospectively or in post hoc analysis) [31–33]:

Dabigatran 150 mg twice daily (TD) if creatinine clearance > 50 ml/min, 110 mg TD if CrCl between 30 and 50. In the USA, the FDA approved 150 mg TD if CrCl >30 and 75 mg TD if ClCr 30–15. Do not use in association with dronedarone; reduce dose if concomitant verapamil is used.
Rivaroxaban 20 mg once daily or 15 mg if CrCl 49–30 ml/min.
Apixaban 5 mg TD or 2.5 mg TD if two or more risk factors for bleeding: age <80 years, weight <60 kg, creatinine >1.5 mg/dl.
Time to peak action is around 3 h for all three.

Valvular AF carries a very high risk per se and must always be treated with VKAs. NOACs were not tested or resulted inferior to VKAs in this setting [5, 34].

For patients with nonvalvular AF, a number of risk stratification schemes have been proposed, the mostly recommended [1, 5] being the CHA2DS2-VASc scoring system [35] (Table 5.1). As chronic therapy, anticoagulation is not indicated for score = 0, indicated for score ≥2, recommended for score = 1 by European guidelines [4], while US guidelines [5] indicate alternatively oral anticoagulants, aspirin or no antithrombotic treatment (Class IIb). We favour oral anticoagulation for patients with score = 1 unless at risk of bleeding.

Any type of AF (paroxysmal, persistent, permanent) carries a similar risk of stroke, so anticoagulation should be chosen regardless of AF type. Atrial flutter has shown to have similar thromboembolic risk as AF and should be managed the same way.

All patients with AF >48 h duration (including those with CHA2DS2-VASc score = 0) candidate to cardioversion must be adequately anticoagulated for at least

Table 5.1 CHA2DS2-VASc scoring system

Acronym	Risk parameter	CHA2DS2VASc score	Stroke rate (%/year)
C	Cardiac failure or dysfunction	0	0
H	Hypertension	1	1.3
A (2)	Age >75	2	2.2
D	Diabetes	3	3.2
S (2)	Stroke/TIA or thromboembolism	4	4
V	Vascular disease	5	6.7
A	Age 65–74	6	9.8
Sc	Sex category (female)	7	9.6
		8	6.7
		9	15.2

Based on Lip et al. [35]
One point is assigned to each parameter except for Age >75 and Stroke whom 2 points are assigned

the three preceding weeks before the procedure, unless intraatrial thrombus has been ruled out by TEE or in case of rare emergency situations and continued on anticoagulation for at least 4 weeks afterwards. Lifelong anticoagulation is indicated for patients at high risk of stroke or AF recurrence.

For patients with AF onset <48 h, current guidelines [4, 5, 10] indicate cardioversion without previous anticoagulation, as former studies demonstrated low embolic complications (0.8 % stroke at 30 days in the study of Weigner et al. [36]). Some concern has raised as it was demonstrated that 4–14 % of these patients had an intraatrial thrombus on transoesophageal echocardiography [37, 38], and ESC 2010 guidelines [4] recommend to start anticoagulation with UFH or LMWH before cardioversion even for AF lasting <48 h. In high-risk patients, heparin therapy has to be followed by long-term oral anticoagulation (class I recommendation), while in patients with no risk factors, heparin therapy may be considered only pericardioversion (IIb, level C recommendation), but this latter recommendation is not evidence based. The 2014 AHA/ACC/HRS guidelines [5] make similar recommendations on use of peri- and postcardioversion antithrombotic therapy, adding the option to use NOACs for the purpose (Class I recommendation). In this context, also a recent European Expert Consensus [28] agrees with the use of NOACs with a class IIa recommendation. A recent large cohort study [39] on 7660 cardioversions of AF lasting <48 h supports the recommendation of prolonged anticoagulation in high-risk patients after CV: without anticoagulation, thromboembolic risk resulted 0.7 % at 30 days. Risk factors were age, heart failure, diabetes, and female gender (elements of CHA2DS2-VASc score system). Patients without risk factors experienced a very low complication rate of 0.2 %, whereas those with multiple risk factors had a thromboembolic risk approaching 10 %.

For patients with AF lasting >48 h or of unknown origin with no risk factors (CHA2DS2-VASc=0), anticoagulation is not advised unless a delayed cardioversion is planned.

6. *Decision for cardiologist consultation or hospitalisation*

Consultation with a cardiologist should be requested for:

- Unstable patients (hypotension, angina, heart failure)
- Patients with known significant cardiac disease
- If significant underlying heat disease is suggested by objective findings, laboratory data or diagnostic testing
- If rate or rhythm control has not been achieved
- If cardiovascular complications have occurred as consequence of antiarrhythmic or rate control therapy
- If cardioversion preceded by TEE is the choice
- If Brugada pattern emerges on ECG after pharmacological cardioversion

Most of these patients will also require hospitalisation, as well as patients with concomitant acute illness (sepsis, pneumonia, pulmonary embolism, etc.).

5.3   What Cardiologists Should Know

"Pill-in-the-pocket approach": useful treatment strategy for patients with no or minimal heart disease, no conduction disturbances and infrequent but prolonged and well tolerated AF recurrences. Patients have to take orally 200–300 mg flecainide or 450–600 mg propafenone (the higher dosage for weight >70 kg). This approach should be prescribed by a cardiologist after full diagnostic workup (and therefore in the author's opinion avoided in first diagnosed AF) and must first be tested in the ED for safety and efficacy before it can be used at home. If this strategy is the choice, the cardiologist should specify this indication on his written evaluation of the patient so that instructions can be promptly be followed in the ED for the first test treatment. In the original article by Alboni et al., [40] rapid 1:1 flutter complicated only 1 case (0.6 %), so ESC 2010 guidelines [4] recommend this strategy as it was described, but AHA/AC/HRS 2014 [5] and CCS 2010 [41] guidelines recommend addition of beta blocker or nondihydropyridine calcium channel blocker to avoid this side effect. This strategy should not be used for patients with AFL.

Patients already on chronic antiarrhythmic therapy may present to the ED with relapsing acute onset AF. If cardioversion is judged to be the choice, we suggest electrical CV as first choice. Alternatively, pharmacological cardioversion (PCV) with the same antiarrhythmic agent administered intravenously at reduced dose can be performed although there is little evidence in literature. In our centre, it has been common practice for more than a decade to use flecainide or propafenone half dose bolus (1 mg/kg in 10 min) on top of chronic therapy with the same agents or intravenous amiodarone with conventional dosages and infusion rates on top of chronic amiodarone therapy, after checking for contraindications. We have not yet experienced significant side effects. Patients are discharged on the same antiarrhythmic agent, even at higher dose, as single or few AF relapses should not be interpreted as treatment failures if the antiarrhythmic burden is lowered on medication. We advise in general against the use of different antiarrhythmic drugs on top of chronic antiarrhythmic drug therapy although limited experience on intravenous ibutilide in patients taking amiodarone, propafenone or flecainide seems safe [42, 43].

Coronary artery disease and atrial fibrillation are often associated diseases [7] and share common risk factors. AF may complicate myocardial infarction in about 18 % [44] and is frequently associated with severe LV damage and heart failure. Fast ventricular rate contributes to increased myocardial damage and heart failure, requiring prompt treatment. Adequate rate control can be obtained preferably by administration of beta blockers (uniformly class I recommendation by ESC 2010, AHA/ACC/HRS 2014, ESC 2012 STEMI guidelines [4, 5, 45]) or in alternative nondihydropyridine calcium antagonists (class IIa in ESC 2010; class IIb in AHA/HRS/ACC 2014; class I in ESC STEMI 2012), in patients who do not display HF or haemodynamic instability. In patients with associated severe left ventricular dysfunction, or signs and symptoms of heart failure, rate control is more safely achieved with i.v. amiodarone or i.v. digoxin (class I in ESC STEMI 2012 [45]; Class IIb in AHA/ACC/HRS 2014 [5]), also in association [45]. Urgent electrical cardioversion should be considered in patients presenting with atrial fibrillation and intractable ischaemia or haemodynamic instability [45].

Pharmacologic cardioversion should be considered if ischemic trigger has resolved with amiodarone being the agent of choice [45].

A still yet unsolved issue is the significance of two common findings, *mildly elevated troponin I (TnI) levels or ST depression* on ECG in the absence of overt acute coronary syndromes (ACS). It is common practice in the EDs to check troponin levels in patients presenting with AF even after excluding primary diagnosis of acute coronary syndrome (76 % of 662 patients in the study of Gupta et al. [46]). The prevalence of mildly positive TnI tests in acute AF patients without evident ACS varies from 9 [47] to 44 % [46]. Troponin I elevation predicts increased the risk of death [48, 49] or MI [46, 48] in the long term. This seems true in the acute setting for minor TnI elevations (detectable but subthreshold) as well as for positive TnI tests (with the higher the value the higher the risk [48]), but also in more chronic AF settings [49]). Troponin elevation is associated with older age, CAD risk factors, known CAD disease, creatinine elevation and ventricular rate but not with angina or ischemic ST depression [46, 28].

It is known that TnI elevations can occur also in the absence of significant coronary stenoses probably because of supply–demand mismatch or atrial–ventricular stretch [46]. Moreover, it has to be taken into account that troponin levels may be elevated for other reasons in acute AF patients (79 % in the study of Meshkat et al. [50] including demand-related rise in 36 %, congestive heart failure in 29 %, renal failure in 17 %, sepsis in 14 % and pneumonia in 2 %).

TnI elevation leads to increased prescription of diagnostic tests for CAD which demonstrated mild diagnostic yield (absent in the study of Gupta et al. [46], useful leading to threefold coronary revascularisation rate and better outcome in the study of Conti et al. [47]). Although these studies confirm that biomarkers seem useful for improving risk prediction in AF, the link between AF and coronary artery disease needs additional investigation.

ECG changes suggesting ischemia (ST segment depression) even in the absence of angina or troponin elevations are also frequent. The positive predictive value for significant CAD varies from 31 [51] to 50 % [52]. Pradhan et al. [51] observed a strong correlation between grade of ST depression and ventricular rate. In their series, the percentages of positive results for diagnostic tests for CAD did not differ significantly between patients with (31 %) or without (21 %) ST depression during AF, so in conclusion, they stated that ST depression during AF is a prevalently rate-related phenomenon.

Absence of ECG changes resulted highly reassuring in the study of Tsigkas et al. [52] (only 4 % prevalence of CAD). In the series of Androulakis et al. [53], the prevalence of ST depression during fast FA was 32.5 %, and non-invasive diagnostic tests performed quite well in identifying patients with CAD.

So what to do in the presence of TnI elevation or new "ischemic" ECG changes during rapid AF?

- *Negative TnI* and *no ECG changes* do not require further investigation.
- *Mildly positive TnI values or ECG changes* should be evaluated in a polyparametric context which accounts for risk factors and cardiac comorbidities.
  - *Lower-risk* patients may be discharged after 12-24 h in an observation unit if stable and troponin descending, possibly after an echocardiogram and non-invasive provocative test for CAD (otherwise these tests should be arranged shortly after as outpatients).
  - *Higher-risk* patients should be admitted.

Heart failure (HF) and AF are strongly associated diseases and can interact to promote their perpetuation as onset of AF can worsen symptoms in patients with HF. These patients should be managed according to clinical severity. If markedly compromised (pulmonary oedema), they should be cardioverted if there is no prompt response to rate control (amiodarone or digoxin are agents of choice) [4]. If clinical presentation is less severe and AF duration is less than 48 h, pharmacological cardioversion with amiodarone or ECV can be considered as alternative to rate control strategy. For rate control purposes, cautious use of beta blockers in patients with systolic heart failure (or diltiazem if HF with preserved EF) can be considered (AHA/ACC/HRS 2014 class I recommendation) [5].

Conversely, worsened HF can promote a rapid ventricular response in permanent AF. These patients usually do not respond to cardioversion and rate control is as well more difficult to achieve. The mainstay of therapy in this setting should be aimed to optimise HF treatment.

Patients may present with newly detected HF in the presence of AF with a rapid ventricular response. These should be presumed to have a rate-related cardiomyopathy, with the arrhythmia being a potentially reversible cause of HF [54]. In this situation, two options can be considered: (1) rate control and re-evaluation for EF improvement and (2) rhythm control, which common practice is to initiate amiodarone and cardiovert in the patient electrically at least 3 weeks later [54]. In our clinic, we try to pursue a more rapid rhythm control strategy for patients with suspected tachycardiomyopathy which consists in performing TEE after clinical stabilisation with HF medications, rate control and anticoagulation. If no thrombus is detected, the patient receives a 24 h amiodarone infusion after which ECV is performed and followed by oral loading dose of amiodarone.

AF in Pre-excitation If very rapid and unstable, urgent ECV should be performed [4, 5, 9]. If heart rate is not too high and the arrhythmia is well tolerated, it can be cardioverted with intravenous flecainide, propafenone, ibutilide and procainamide. The same agents are effective of rate control [4, 5, 20]. Drugs acting on the AV node, like calcium channel blockers, digitalis and adenosine, are contraindicated, because conduction over the accessory pathway is favoured and the rate transmission to the ventricle may become very rapid potentially inducing ventricular fibrillation. Amiodarone has recently been defined as harmful in the AHA/ACC/HRS 2014 guidelines [5], whereas ESC guidelines 2010 [4] recommend it class I for rate control. Beta blockers are contraindicated according to ESC guidelines 2010 [4] but might be used with caution according to the AHA/ACC/HRS 2014 guidelines [5].

5.4 A Possible Algorithm/Pathway for Diagnosis and Treatment

The management of patients with AF depends on their clinical presentation which may be unstable (Fig 5.8), stable with AF onset < 48 hours (Fig. 5.9) or stable with AF onset > 48 hours/undefined onset (Fig 5.10).

If cardioversion is the choice, check potassium levels (unless emergent ECV is necessary) and correct it if necessary proceeding. If patient is on chronic digoxin therapy, plasma level should be checked (ECV is contraindicated in case of intoxication).

In general, ECV is more effective than pharmacological cardioversion (PCV) and requires less time, but greater organisational efforts.

SR is achieved in about 90 % with ECV and 70 % with PCV [55]. If PCV fails, ECV restores SR in the majority of cases. On the contrary, if AF relapses immediately (IRAF) after ECV, the use of an antiarrhythmic agent before repeat CVE enhances the probability of maintaining SR. If AF does not convert to sinus rhythm with ECV (no or a maximum single sinus beat achieved, as defined by ESC 2010 guidelines [4]), the patient can be pretreated with ibutilide (1 mg over 10 min) which lowers defibrillation threshold and facilitates greatly achievement of SR on repeat ECV [56].

Pharmacologic cardioversion is little effective after 7 days of AF onset; therefore, in this case, ECV is preferred.

Atrial flutter poorly responds to antiarrhythmic drugs except for ibutilide; therefore, ECV should be first choice. If propafenone or flecainide are used for AFL conversion, slowing of atrial rate occurs, which sometimes can conduct faster to the ventricles (from usual 2:1 to 1:1 conduction), often with conduction aberrancy (Fig. 5.6). The result is a very rapid, frequently untolerated arrhythmia which should be electrically cardioverted. So if these agents are used for treatment of AFL, co-administration of rate control drugs is advised. The same phenomenon may occur when flecainide or propafenone is used for conversion of AF, as in some cases AF organizes into AFL ("IC flutter"). In rare cases of patients treated with these agents, an electrocardiographic "Brugada pattern" may become evident (coved-type ST elevation in at least one lead from V1 to V3). These patients should undergo cardiologic consultation before eventual discharge.

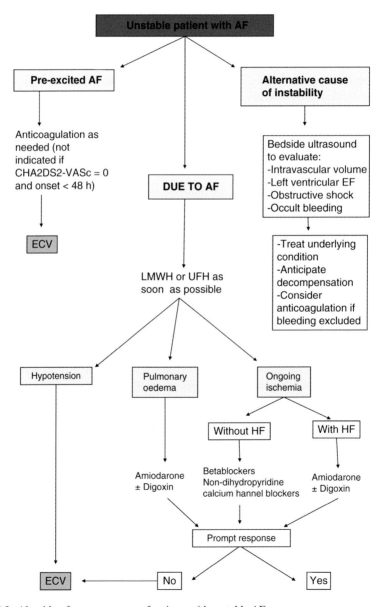

Fig. 5.8 Algorithm for management of patients with unstable AF

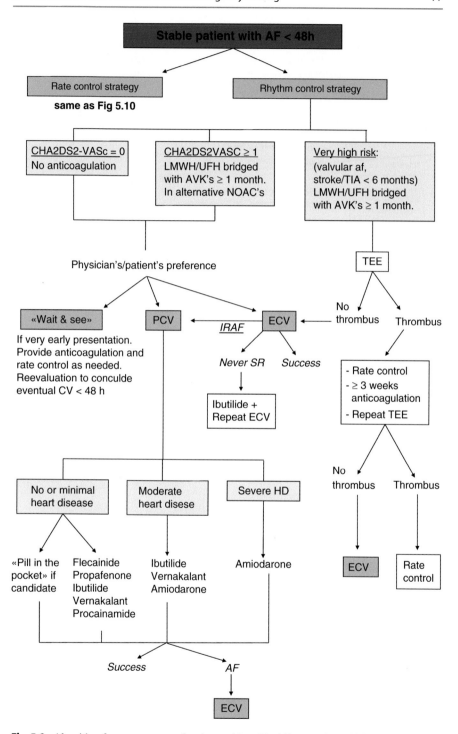

Fig. 5.9 Algorithm for management of patients with stable AF presenting <48 h from onset

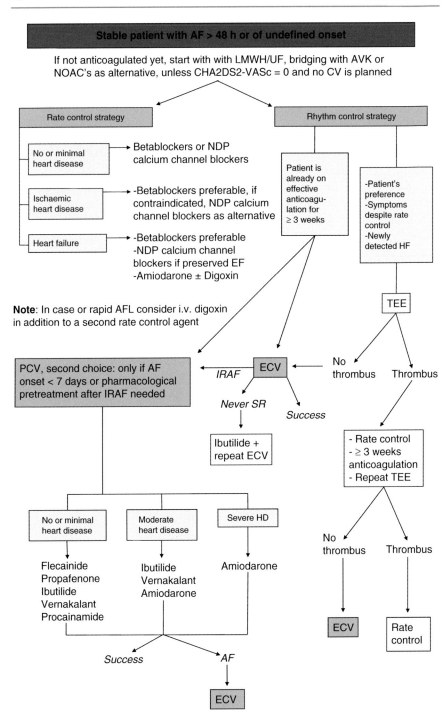

Fig. 5.10 Algorithm for management of patients with stable AF presenting >48 h from onset

A patient who has undergone pharmacological cardioversion should be monitored for a period afterwards (usually half of the drugs elimination's half life) to rule out bradycardia, AV block or ventricular proarrhythmia or hypotension, before discharge. If a patient has been electrically cardioverted, at least 3 h of monitoring is needed [4].

5.4.1 Electrical Cardioversion

Sedation can be provided by different professionals, based on competence, organisation and therapy used. Emergency physicians are involved in the great majority throughout the world for AF cardioversion in the ED. Less often, cardiologists or anaesthesiologists supervise the procedure [21].

A number of medications can be used, like benzodiazepines, narcotics and propofol, alone or in combination. *Midazolam*, a benzodiazepine with a short half-life is gaining increased diffusion because of its pharmacodynamics, wide therapeutic range and availability of a reversal agent (flumazenil). In the two major series [57, 58], adequate sedation was achieved in nearly all patients and no serious complications were observed. Usually, initial bolus doses of 0.01–01 mg/kg are used (the higher ones when the agent is used alone), which may be followed by repeated boli. Mean total dosage used throughout major studies on the use of midazolam as single agent was around 10 mg [59]. *Propofol* is another popular agent for sedation as it has an even more rapid onset of action and washout. On the other hand, it has a greater potential for hypotension and respiratory depression. It is used at dosages of 1–2.5 mg/kg [60].

The procedure can be performed with older monophasic or newer biphasic defibrillators. The latter are more effective with lower energy requirements [61]. The device is connected to the body by a couple of adhesive pads or a couple of hand-held paddles.

Four pad positions are currently used: anterolateral, anteroposterior, anterior–left infrascapular and anterior–right infrascapular. They are equally effective to treat atrial or ventricular arrhythmias [62]. If paddles are used (anterolateral position), the operator should press firmly, the optimal force being 8 kg. If the patient has an implantable cardioverter defibrillator (or a pacemaker), anteroposterior or anterolateral locations are acceptable and the nearest pad or paddle should be positioned at least 8 cm away from the device [63]. After the procedure, the device should be interrogated and evaluated to ensure normal function [4]. The DC shock must be synchronised to the R wave to avoid the risk of inducing ventricular fibrillation.

The recommended initial biphasic energy dose for ECV of adult atrial fibrillation is 120–200 Joules (J), whereas for atrial flutter, 50–100 J is usually sufficient. If CV fails, energy should be stepwise increased or the position of the pads changed. For monophasic defibrillators, cardioversion should start at 200 J (100 J for AFL) [10, 62, 63].

Complications They are more often related to arrhythmias, usually transient asystole or bradycardia (0.9 % in the acute CV setting of the Fin CV study [39]).

Pre-cardioversion antiarrhythmic therapy, rate control therapy or slow ventricular rate did not predict bradyarrhythmias, whereas older age, female sex or unsuccessful CV did.

Thromboembolic complications are rare but not negligible if patients are adequately stratified and treated.

Ventricular arrhythmias are exceptional as are episodes of pulmonary oedema.

Complications can rarely be related to sedation like hypotension and prolonged respiratory arrest but are managed with conventional support (fluids and manual ventilation) in the great majority.

5.4.2 Drugs for Rhythm and Rate Control

- Note1: not all drugs or formulations for i.v. or oral use are available in all countries.
- Note 2: for rate and rhythm control drugs, dosages and infusion protocols usually vary between the different guidelines [1, 4, 5, 10, 20, 41]. If there is agreement between sources (or with little variations), one protocol is reported, which also corresponds to the author's practice. If there are marked differences, alternative protocols are mentioned.

5.4.2.1 Rhythm Control Drugs

Flecainide Sodium channel blocker with quite rapid action restores SR in 67–92 % in 6 h. Dosage: 2 mg/kg i.v. over 10 min. Ideal agent for patients with no or minimal heart disease. Avoid in patients with ischaemic heart disease, left ventricular dysfunction, intraventricular conduction delay or Brugada Syndrome. Risks are ventricular proarrhythmia, AV block and electromechanical dissociation. When used for conversion of AFL, 1:1 conduction may ensue with rapid ventricular rate if no rate control agent has been associated. In some countries (USA), approved only for oral use. In this case, 200–300 mg is administered orally (the same dose as the "pill-in-the-pocket" approach), AHA/ACC/HRS 2014 [5] and CCS 2010 [64] guidelines recommending administration of a beta blocker or calcium channel blocker before.

Propafenone Similar properties, indications and efficacy as for flecainide. Dosage: 2 mg/kg i.v. over 10 min. Avoid also in severe COPD because of its weak noncompetitive beta blocking property. In the USA available orally only: administrate 450–600 mg preceded by AV node-blocking agent as above.

Procainamide Sodium channel blocker. Dosage: 15–17 mg/kg i.v. over 1 h with conversion rate around 60 %. Very popular in Canada. Recommended for AF conversion in stable patients in CCS guidelines 2010 [64]. Causes transient hypotension in 5 %.

Amiodarone Multichannel blocker, also with beta- and calcium channel blocking activity if used intravenously. Prolongs prevalently refractoriness in chronic use. Dosage: 5 mg/kg in 1 h, then 50 mg/h for 24 h (ESC 2010 [4]) or 150 mg in 10 min, then 1 mg/min for 6 h, then 0.5 mg/min for 18 h (AHA/ACC/HRS 2014 [5]).

Amiodarone should be diluted in 5 % glucose solution (otherwise there is a risk of crystallisation of the solution). It restores SR with delayed action but similar efficacy as flecainide and propafenone at 12–24 h. It has also significant rate-slowing properties. It is the agent of choice for patients with severe heart disease for both purposes of cardioversion and rate control. Contraindicated in hyperthyroidism, avoid if possible in patients with severe COPD and hypothyroidism. Most common acute side effects are hypotension (especially if infusion is too fast) and phlebitis (the longer the infusion lasts, the more probable).

Ibutilide Rapid-acting agent, prolongs repolarisation. Dosage: 1 mg i.v. over 10 min, if unsuccessful, repeat after 10 min same dose. AF conversion rate is around 50 % with time to conversion about 30 min. Best available conversion agent for AFL. It carries a considerable risk of QTc prolongation and torsades de pointes (4 %). Patients should be monitored for a minimum of 4 h after. Some authors suggest pretreatment with 1–2 g MgSO₄ to lower the proarrhythmic risk. Contraindicated if patients are hypotensive, have manifest congestive heart failure, have very low EF (<30 %) and hypokalemic or if QTc >440 ms. Pretreatment with 1 mg over 10 min facilitates great ECV in patients who failed it before.

Dofetilide Prolongs repolarization. Has been mostly studied in the setting of persistent AF. A response may take days or weeks, and therefore it is not an ideal agent in the ED setting. Mentioned and recommended class I only in 2014 AHA/ACC/HRS guidelines [5]. Dosages: 500 mcg BID if creatinine clearance (CrCl) >60, 250 mcg BID if 40–60, 125 mcg BID if 20–40. Do not use if CrCl under 20 ml/min. Do not initiate treatment out of hospital (risk of torsades de pointes).

Vernakalant Fast-acting atrial selective multichannel blocker with conversion rate around 50 % and median time to conversion about 10 min. Dosage: 3 mg/kg i.v. over 10 min, followed, if unsuccessful, by second infusion of 2 mg/kg i.v. over 10 min after 15. Contraindicated in hypotensive patients (<100 mmHg), NYHA 3–4 heart failure, FE <35 %, ACS in the last 30 days, severe aortic stenosis and QTc >440 ms.

5.4.2.2 Rate Control Drugs

Beta blockers Very effective, first choice in acute coronary syndrome or heart failure patients (avoid or use with extreme caution in acute decompensation). Do not use in severe COPD and pre-excitation syndrome. Metoprolol, atenolol and propranolol can be used intravenously and orally and are therefore the most useful for acute and chronic treatment. Esmolol is available intravenously only and is frequently used in the intensive care setting. Other beta blockers like bisoprolol or carvedilol are available for oral administration only and can be used if rate control is not too urgent and for chronic therapy.

- Metoprolol: 2.5–5 mg i.v. in 2 min every 5 min up to three doses (max 15 mg), oral maintenance dose 50–200 mg/day
- Atenolol: 2.5 mg i.v. at a rate of 1 mg/min to be repeated at intervals of 5 min up to a maximum of 10 mg
- Propranolol 1 mg i.v. over 1 min up to three doses at 2 min intervals, oral maintenance dose 30–160 mg/day
- Esmolol 0.5 mg/kg i.v. bolus over 1 min, then 50–300 mcg/kg/min i.v.

Nondihydropyridine (NDP) and Calcium Channel Blockers (Diltiazem, Verapamil) Very effective, diltiazem is the less inotropic negative and hypotensive of the two. Avoid in heart failure patients (with the exception of HF with preserved systolic function if not acutely decompensated) and pre-excitation syndrome.

- Verapamil: 0.075–0.15 mg/kg i.v. bolus over 2 min, may repeat 10 mg bolus after 30 min if uneffective, then 0.005 mg/kg/min infusion [5]. Oral maintenance dose 160–360 mg/day
- Diltiazem 0.25 mg/kg i.v. bolus over 2 min, may give a second dose of 0.35 mg/kg, then 5–15 mg/h infusion. Oral maintenance dose 180–360 mg/day

Amiodarone Usually second-line agent. It is well tolerated in critically ill patients where it can be the first choice.

Digoxin Usually a second-line agent with moderate and delayed efficacy on rate control. When used intravenously, onset of action takes 1 h and peak rate-slowing activity is reached at 6 h. It is first-line agent in patients with acute heart failure. Due to its vagomimetic activity, it tends to transform atrial flutter in fibrillation (about 25 %, personal observation) so it turns out very helpful in rate control for flutter, which is harder to achieve than for AF. In the author's practice, digoxin is used as first-line agent, associated with another rate control drug when fixed. 2:1 AV conduction with rapid ventricular rate is present. Avoid in moderate or severe renal failure due to risk of intoxication.

Dosage 0.25–0.5 mg i.v. with repeat dosing, maximum 1.5 mg/24 h. Oral maintenance dose 0.0625–0.25 mg/day

5.5 Indications for Hospitalisation, Follow-Up and Referral

Hospitalisation should be in general considered for patients with AF and severe symptoms (heart failure, severe angina, syncope), when a significant heart disease is suspected, important comorbidities are present, symptoms are not properly controlled (failed cardioversion or rate control) or if complications occur during first approach treatment.

Decision algorithms like RED-AF [65] and AFFORD [66] have recently developed for predicting 30 days adverse events in AF patients presenting to ED with AF. Nomograms contain many clinical predictors and points are assigned to each predictor. Adverse events vary from ED return visit for recurrent AF to death, through different grades of severity. The AFFORD [66] model fared well in risk prediction and in the identification of patients at very low risk which the authors stated could be safely discharged after cardioversion or adequate rate control, but these were only 17 % of the total. This still poses the problem of the acceptable risk threshold for indicating hospitalisation (e.g. is it worth to hospitalise a patient to avoid return visit for AF relapse? Is stroke preventable by hospitalisation if patient is properly anticoagulated also at home?). Furthermore, the same authors admit that the effect of hospitalising ED patients with acute AF on short-term adverse events remains unanswered [65] (RED-AF). Uncertainties on hospitalisation criteria are still reflected by the wide discrepancy of the discharge rate after successful CV: 85 % in Canada, 76 % in Australasia, 48 % in the USA and 27 % in the UK [21].

In the absence of obvious severe presentation or comorbidities, careful individual judgement on high-risk features should be performed to guide this decision.

It should be stressed that new-onset AF carries a worse prognosis [7, 18]. In the study of Miyasaka et al. [67], hazard ratio for mortality risk was 9.6 within the first 4 months and 1.7 thereafter, compared with age- and gender-matched general population. The main reason is thought to be that AF complicates underlying conditions with poor prognosis like cardiovascular diseases or malignancies. As a consequence, patients with first episode should undergo a rapid medical workup which can be done of course during hospitalisation, but alternatively, if there is no clinical instability, on outpatient basis. In order to favour the latter strategy, diagnostic pathways which include evaluation by cardiologist and other professionals as well as diagnostic testings should be defined locally and be easily accessible, which is unfortunately not always the case and gives reason for the high percentage of hospitalisation of AF patients in some countries [23].

Follow-up of AF patients should be individualised and take into account symptomatic status, comorbidities (which should be followed up as specifically needed), antiarrhythmic treatment, thromboprophylaxis and complications. Visits should be usually performed by the primary care physician or a cardiologist.

Asymptomatic patients in sinus rhythm without medications and comorbidities do not need a structured follow-up, and a periodic self-check of pulse regularity should be recommended.

Patients on antiarrhythmic or on rate control medications should get an ECG 1 week after beginning or up-titration of therapy to check for efficacy and proarrhythmic complications and a visit every 6–12 months.

At every follow-up visit, the following issues should be reassessed:

- Effectiveness of symptom control either while pursuing rate or rhythm control strategy
- Need for antithrombotic therapy, re-evaluation of risks and benefits
- Optimization of therapy for comorbidities
- Lifestyle counselling and check for adequate compliance

Furthermore, in relation to individual therapy, there may be a need for periodical lab tests (e.g. thyroid function for patients on amiodarone, liver function for patients on dronedarone, blood count and renal function for patients using novel anticoagulants, etc.).

Echocardiography should be performed as recommended for underlying structural heart disease or in case of worsening symptoms despite apparent achievement of rate or rhythm control. Holter recording may be needed for assessment of adequate rate control or if proarrhythmia is suspected. An exercise stress test can help to adjust rate control medications in active patients with permanent AF who complain uncontrolled palpitations during exercise.

Referral to a cardiologist *is generally indicated for patients with a first AF episode.* A possible exception is older patients with asymptomatic AF with adequate rate control. Basic screening examinations like laboratory tests, thyroid function and echocardiography should be arranged before referral. Other reasons for referral to a cardiologist are inadequate rhythm control strategy (ineffective or not tolerated antiarrhythmic medications), ineffective rate control strategy (inadequate rate control or poor quality of life despite adequate rate control) and evaluation for radiofrequency ablation.

References

1. Camm AJ, Lip GYH, De Caterina R, et al. 2012 focused update of the ESC guidelines for the management of atrial fibrillation. An update of the 2010 ESC guidelines for the management of atrial fibrillation. Eur Heart J. 2012;33:2719–47.
2. Santini M, De Ferrari GM, Pandozi C, et al. Atrial fibrillation requiring urgent medical care. Approach and outcome in the various departments of admission. Data from the atrial Fibrillation/flutter Italian Registry (FIRE). Ital Heart J. 2004;5:205–13.
3. Coll-Vinent B, Martìn A, Malagòn F, et al. Stroke prophylaxis in atrial fibrillation: searching for management improvement opportunities in the emergency department: the HERMES-AF Study. Ann Emerg Med. 2015;65:1–12.
4. Camm JA, Kirchhof P, Lip GYH, et al. Guidelines for the management of atrial fibrillation. The task force for the management of atrial fibrillation of the European Society of Cardiology (ESC). Eur Heart J. 2010;31:2369–429.
5. January CT, Wann LS, Alpert JS, et al. 2014 AHA/ACC/HRS Guideline for the management of patients with atrial fibrillation. A report of the American College of Cardiology/American Heart Association and the Heart Rhythm Society task force of practical guidelines. J Am Coll Cardiol. 2014;64:2246–80.
6. Thrall G, Lane D, Carrol D, et al. Quality of life in patients with atrial fibrillation: a systematic review. Am J Med. 2006;119:448e1–448e19.
7. Nieuwlaat R, Cappucci A, Camm JA, et al. Atrial fibrillation management: a prospective survey in ESC member countries. Eur Heart J. 2005;26:2422–34.
8. Oishi ML, Xing S. Atrial fibrillation: management strategies in the emergency department. Emerg Med Pract. 2013;15:1–26.
9. Neumar R, Otto CW, Link MS, et al. Adult advanced cardiovascular life support: part 8. 2010 American Heart Association guidelines for cardiopulmonary resuscitation and emergency cardiovascular care. Circulation. 2010;122 Suppl 3:S 729–767.
10. Verma A, Cairns JA, Mitchell LB, et al. 2014 focused update of the Canadian Cardiovascular Society guidelines for the management of atrial fibrillation. Can J Cardiol. 2014;30:1114–30.
11. Nabauer M, Gerth A, Limbourg T, et al. The registry of german competence network on atrial fibrillation: patient characteristics and initial management. Europace. 2009;11:423–34.
12. Buccelletti F, Carroccia A, Marsiliani D, et al. Utility of routine thyroid-stimulation hormone determination in new-onset atrial fibrillation in the ED. Am J Emerg Med. 2011;29:1158–62.
13. Bellone A, Etteri M, Vettorello M, et al. Cardioversion of acute atrial fibrillation in the emergency department: a prospective randomised trial. Emerg Med J. 2012;29:188–91.
14. Healey JS, Parkash R, Pollak T, et al. Canadian Cardiovascular Society guidelines 2010: etiology and initial investigations. Can J Cardiol. 2011;27:31–7.

15. Atzema C, Lam KM, Young C, et al. Patients with atrial fibrillation and an alternative primary diagnosis in the emergency department: a description of their characteristics and outcomes. Acad Emerg Med. 2013;10:193–9.
16. Scheuermeier FX, Pourvali R, Rowe BH, et al. Emergency department patients with atrial fibrillation or flutter and acute underlying medical illness may not benefit from attempts to control rate or rhythm. Ann Emerg Med. 2015;65:511–22.
17. Wyse DG, Waldo AL, Di Marco JP, The atrial fibrillation follow-up investigation of rhythm management (AFFIRM) investigators, et al. A comprison of rate control and rhythm control in patients with atrial fibrillation. N Engl J Med. 2002;347:1825–33.
18. Camm JA, Breithardt G, Crijns H, et al. Real-life observations of clinical outcomes with rhythm- and rate control therapies for atrial fibrillation. RECORDAF (registry on cardiac rhythm disorders assessing the control of atrial fibrillation). J Am Coll Cardiol. 2011;58:493–501.
19. Alam M, Jamaluddin Bandeali S, Shahzad SA, et al. Real–life global survey evaluating patients with atrial fibrillation (REALISE-AF): results of an international observational registry. Expert Rev Cardiovasc Ther. 2012;10:283–91.
20. Raviele A, Disertori M, Alboni P, et al. Linee guida AIAC per la gestione ed il trattamento della fibrillazione atriale. Aggiornamento 2013. G Ital Cardiol. 2013;14:215–40.
21. Rogenstein C, Kelly A-M, Mason S, et al. An international view of how recent onset atrial fibrillation is treated in the emergency department. Acad Emerg Med. 2012;19:1255–60.
22. Stiell IG, Birnie D. Clinical controversies: in a vacuum of good evidence, rhythm control is the sensible option for patients with symptomatic recent onset atrial fibrillation or flutter. Ann Emerg Med. 2011;57:31–2.
23. Cohn BG, Keim SM, Yealy DM. Is emergency department cardioversion of recent-onset atrial fibrillation safe and effective? J Emerg Med. 2013;45:117–27.
24. Stiell IG, Clement CM, Perry JJ, et al. Association of the "Ottawa aggressive protocol" with rapid discharge of emergency department patients with recent-onset atrial fibrillation or flutter. CJEM. 2010;12:181–91.
25. Danias PG, Caulfield TA, Weigner MJ, et al. Likelihood of spontaneous conversion of atrial fibrillation to sinus rhythm. J Am Coll Cardiol. 1998;31:588–92.
26. Vinson DR, Hoehn T, Graber DJ, et al. Managing emergency department patients with recent-onset atrial fibrillation. J Emerg Med. 2012;42:139–48.
27. Decker WW, Smars PA, Vaidjanathan L, et al. A prospective randomized trial of an emergency department observation unit for acute onset atrial fibrillation. Emerg Med. 2008;52:322–8.
28. De Caterina R, Husted S, Wallentin L, et al. Parenteral anticoagulants in heart disease: current status and perspectives (section II). Position paper of the ESC working group on thrombosis – task force on anticoagulants in heart disease. Thromb Haemost. 2013;109:769–86.
29. Klein AL, Jasper SE, Katz WE, et al. The use of enoxaparin compared with unfractionated heparin for short-term antithrombotic therapy in atrial fibrillation patients undergoing transoesophageal echocardiography–guided cardioversion: assessment of cardioversion using transoesophageal echocardiography (ACUTE) II randomized multicenter study. Eur Heart J. 2006;27:2858–65.
30. Stellbrink C, Nixdorff U, Hofmann T, et al. Safety and efficacy of enoxaparin compared with unfractionated heparin and oral anticoagulants for prevention of thromboembolic complications in cardioversion with nonvalvular atrial fibrillation: the anticoagulation in cardioversion using enoxaparin (ACE) trial. Circulation. 2004;109:997–1003.
31. Nagarakanti R, Ezekowitz MD, Oldgren J, et al. Dabigatran versus warfarin in patients with atrial fibrillation. An analysis on patients undergoing cardioversion. Circulation. 2011;123:113–36.
32. Cappato R, Ezekowitz MD, Klein AL, et al. Rivaroxaban vs vitamin K antagonists for cardioversion in atrial fibrillation. Eur Heart J. 2014;35:3346–55.
33. Flaker G, Lopes RD, Al-Kahib SM, et al. Efficacy and safety of apixaban after cardioversion for atrial fibrillation. J Am Coll Cardiol. 2014;62:1082–7.

34. Van der Werf F, Brueckmann M, Connolly SJ, et al. A comparison of dabigatran etexilate with warfarin in patients with mechanical heart valves: the randomized, phase II study to evaluate the safety and pharmacokinetics of oral dabigatran etexilate in patients after heart valve replacement (RE-ALIGN). Am Heart J. 2012;163:931–7.
35. Lip GY, Frison L, Halperin J, et al. Identifying patients at risk of stroke despite anticoagulation. Stroke. 2010;41:2731–5.
36. Weigner MJ, Caufield TA, Danias PJ, et al. Risk for clinical thromboembolism associated with conversion to sinus rhythm in patients with atrial fibrillation lasting less than 48 hours. Ann Intern Med. 1997;126:615–20.
37. Kleemann T, Becker T, Strauss M, et al. Prevalence of left atrial thrombus and dense spontaneous echo-contrast in patients with short term atrial fibrillation <48 hours undergoing cardioversion: value of transesophageal echocardiography to guide cardioversion. J Am Soc Echocardiogr. 2009;22:1403–8.
38. Stoddart MF, Dawkins PR, Prince CR, et al. Transesophageal echocardiographic guidance of cardioversion in patients with atrial fibrillation. Am Heart J. 1995;129:1204–15.
39. Airaksinen KEJ, Groeneberg T, Nuotio I, et al. Thromboembolic complications after cardioversion of acute atrial fibrillation. The FinCV (Finnish CardioVersion) Study. J Am Coll Cardiol. 2013;62:1187–92.
40. Alboni P, Botto GL, Baldi N, et al. Outpatient treatment of recent onset atrial fibrillation with the "pill in te pocket" approach. N Engl J Med. 2004;351:2384–91.
41. Gillis AM, Verma A, Talajic M, et al. Canadian Cardiovascular Society guidelines 2010: rate and rhythm control management. Can J Cardiol. 2011;27:47–59.
42. Glatter K, Yang Y, Chatterjee K, et al. Chemical cardioversion of atrial fibrillation or flutter with ibutilide in patients receiving amiodarone therapy. Circulation. 2001;103:253–7.
43. Hongo RH, Themistoclakis S, Raviele A, et al. Use of ibutilide in cardioversion of patients with atrial fibrillation or atrial flutter treated with class IC agents. J Am Coll Cardiol. 2004;44:864–8.
44. Sugiura T, Iwasaka T, Ogawa A, et al. Atrial fibrillation i myocardial infarction. Am J Cardiol. 1985;56:27–9.
45. Steg G, James SK, Atar D, et al. ESC guidelines for the management of acute myocardial infarction presenting with ST-segment elevation. Eur Heart J. 2012;33:2569–619.
46. Gupta K, Pillarisetti J, Biria M, et al. Clinical utility and prognostic significance of measuring troponin I levels in patients presenting to the emergency room with atrial fibrillation. Clin Cardiol. 2014;37:343–9.
47. Conti A, Mariannini Y, Canuti E, et al. Role of masked coronary heart disease in patients with recent onset atrial fibrillation and troponin elevations. Eur J Emerg Med. 2015;22:162–9.
48. Van den Bos E, Constantinescu AA, van Domburg RT, et al. Minor elevations in troponin I are associated with mortality and adverse cardiac events in patients with atrial fibrillation. Eur Heart J. 2011;32:611–7.
49. Hijazi Z, Oldgren J, Andersson U, et al. Cardiac biomarkers are associated with an increased risk of stroke ad death in patients with atrial fibrillation. A randomized evaluation of long-term anticoagulation therapy (RE-LY) substudy. Circulation. 2012;125:1605–16.
50. Meshkat N, Austin E, Moineddin R, et al. Troponin utilization in patients presenting with atrial fibrillation/flutter to the emergency department: retrospective chart review. Int J Emerg Med. 2011;4:25.
51. Pradhan R, Chaudhary A, Donato AA. Predictive accuracy of ST depression during rapid atrial fibrillation in the presence on obstructive coronary artery disease. Am J Emerg Med. 2012;30:1042–7.
52. Tsigkas G, Kopsida G, Xanthoupoulou I, et al. Diagnostic accuracy of electrocardiographic ST segment depression in patients with rapid atrial fibrillation for the prediction of coronary artery disease. Can J Cardiol. 2014;30:920–4.
53. Androulakis A, Aznaouridis KA, Aggeli CJ, et al. Transient ST-segment depression during paroxysms of atrial fibrillation in otherwise normal individuals. J Am Coll Cardiol. 2007;19:1909–13.

54. Yancy CW, Jessup M, Bozkurt B, et al. 2013 ACCF/AHA guideline for the management of heart failure: a report of the American College of Cardiology Foundation/American Heart Association task force on practice guidelines. Circulation. 2013;128:e240–327.
55. Crijns HJGM, Weijs B, Fairley A-M, et al. Contemporary real life cardioversion of atrial fibrillation: results from the multinational RHYTHM-AF study. Int J Cardiol. 2014;172:588–94.
56. Oral H, Souza JJ, Michaud GF, et al. Facilitating electrical cardioversion of atrial fibrillation with ibutilide pretreatment. N Engl J Med. 1999;340:1849–59.
57. Huebner PJ, Gupta S, McClellan I, et al. Simplified cardioversion service with intravenous midazolam. Heart. 2004;90:1447–9.
58. Notarstefano P, Pratola C, Toselli T, et al. Sedation with midazolam for electrical cardioversion. PACE. 2007;30:608–11.
59. Thomas SP, Thakkar J, Kovoor P, et al. Sedation for electrophysiological procedures. PACE. 2014;37:781–90.
60. Wood J. Procedural sedation for cardioversion. Emerg Med J. 2006;23:932–4.
61. Mittal S, Ayati S, Stein KM, et al. Transthoracic cardioversion of atrial fibrillation: comparison of rectilinear biphasic versus damped sine wave monophasic shocks. Circulation. 2000;101:1282–7.
62. Link MS, Atkins DL, Passmann RS, et al. American Heart Association guidelines for cardiopulmonary resuscitation and emergency cardiovascular care. Part 6: electrical therapies. Automated external defibrillators, defibrillation, cardioversion and pacing. Circulation 2010; 2010;122 Suppl 3:S706–19.
63. Deakin DD, Nolan JP, Sunde K, et al. European Resuscitation Council guidelines for resuscitation 2010 Section 3. Electrical therapies: automated external defibrillators, defibrillation, cardioversion and pacing. Resuscitation. 2010;81:1293–304.
64. Stiell IG. Macle L and the CCS Atrial Fibrillation Guidelines Committee: Canadian Cardiovascular Society guidelines 2010: management of recent-onset atrial fibrillation and flutter in the emergency department. Can J Cardiol. 2010;27:38–46.
65. Barret TW, Jenkins CA, Self WH. Validation of the risk estimator decision aid for atrial fibrillation (RED-AF) for predicting 30-day adverse events in emergency department patients with atrial fibrillation. Ann Emerg Med. 2015;65:13–21.
66. Barrett TW, Storrow AB, Jenkins CA, et al. The AFFORD clinical decision aid to identify emergency department patients with atrial fibrillation at low risk for 30-day adverse events. Am J Cardiol. 2015;115:763–70.
67. Miyasaka Y, Barnes ME, Bailey KR, et al. Mortality trends in patients diagnosed with first atrial fibrillation. J Am Coll Cardiol. 2007;49:986–92.

Wide QRS Complex Tachycardia in the Emergency Setting

6

Giuseppe Oreto, Francesco Luzza, Gaetano Satullo,
Antonino Donato, Vincenzo Carbone,
and Maria Pia Calabrò

6.1 Wide QRS Complex Tachycardia

A wide QRS complex tachycardia can be (1) ventricular tachycardia (VT); (2) supraventricular tachycardia (SVT) with bundle branch block that may be either preexisting or due to aberrant conduction, namely, tachycardia-dependent abnormal intraventricular conduction; a further possibility is the effect of some antiarrhythmic drugs that slow down intraventricular conduction, resulting in marked QRS complex widening; and (3) supraventricular tachycardia with conduction of impulses to the ventricles over an accessory pathway (preexcited tachycardia).

In the presence of wide QRS tachycardia, the correct diagnosis is of paramount importance, since the treatment commonly used in SVT is different from that of VT, and some drugs useful in the former (e.g., verapamil) are harmful in the latter [1–3].

The origin of a wide QRS complex tachycardia can be reliably identified using a "holistic" approach, namely, taking into account all of the available items: no single criterion is able to provide a simple and quick solution of the problem in all cases. The available ECG signs are, without any exception, suggestive of ectopy, namely, ventricular origin of the impulses; SVT with aberrant conduction may only be diagnosed by excluding all of the items favoring VT. The recognition of ventricular or supraventricular origin of wide QRS complex tachycardias is not difficult if a

G. Oreto (✉) • F. Luzza • V. Carbone
Department of Clinical and Experimental Medicine, University of Messina,
Messina, Italy
e-mail: goreto@unime.it

G. Satullo • A. Donato
Department of Cardiology, "Papardo" Hospital, Messina, Italy

M.P. Calabrò
Department of Pediatrics, University of Messina, Messina, Italy

© Springer International Publishing Switzerland 2016
M. Zecchin, G. Sinagra (eds.), *The Arrhythmic Patient in the Emergency
Department: A Practical Guide for Cardiologists and Emergency Physicians*,
DOI 10.1007/978-3-319-24328-3_6

detailed analysis is used, taking into account several diagnostic signs: [4–12] the idea that a single quick item can offer an immediate and reliable solution is something of an illusion.

If, despite a complete diagnostic approach, the dilemma cannot be resolved, it is necessary to assume a ventricular origin of the arrhythmia since (1) a wide QRS tachycardia is more likely VT than SVT and (2) it is less dangerous to treat an SVT like it were ventricular in origin than applying to a patient with VT the treatment commonly used for SVTs. In particular, intravenous verapamil should be avoided whenever SVT diagnosis is not certain, since this drug is harmful in some VT patients [1–3].

6.2   General Criteria

6.2.1   Atrioventricular Dissociation

Whenever the electrical activity of the atria is recognizable, two different situations may occur:

1. Atrioventricular (A-V) dissociation
2. Relationship between P waves and QRS complexes.

A-V dissociation demonstrates the ventricular origin of the wide QRS complexes and occurs in a percentage variable from 19 to 70 % of VT cases [5, 6, 10, 11]. Dissociation, however, is often difficult to be diagnosed since in several cases, sinus P waves are not easily recognizable, being simultaneous to QRS complexes or T waves. Moreover, in the presence of atrial fibrillation, A-V dissociation cannot be appreciated. Before excluding, in a wide QRS complexes tachycardia, the presence of P waves independent of QRS complexes, however, one should observe with great attention the configuration of several consecutive complexes in all 12 leads, paying the greatest attention to leads II and V1 (the ones where sinus P waves are usually evident). Aim of this analysis is comparing consecutive complexes searching for slight differences in QRS or T morphology: with this approach it is not rare to discover, in the presence of VT, that in some leads, slight variations in QRS complex or T wave configuration occur. To be sure that such differences express the presence of P waves dissociated from QRS complexes, and superimposed on these, it is necessary to measure the intervals separating the "disturbing" events: in case of A-V dissociation, they are separated from relatively constant intervals, being "long" intervals in multiples of the "short" ones (Fig. 6.1a). When, in contrast, the intervals separating the changes in morphology of T waves and/or QRS complexes are irregular, it is more likely that artifacts, rather than dissociated sinus P waves, are involved (Fig. 6.1b).

The best ECG leads to be analyzed, searching for "dissociated" P waves, are leads II and V1, the ones where sinus P wave voltage is usually relatively high; it is also advisable to observe the leads where the QRS complex and/or the T wave is of

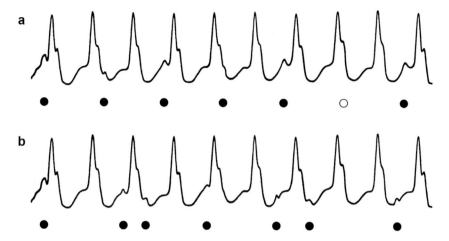

Fig. 6.1 Diagrams (**a**, **b**) show two wide QRS complex tachycardias. In both diagrams, small positive deflections, independent of QRS complexes, are present. In diagram (**a**) these deflections are rhythmic and separated by constant intervals; whenever a deflection is invisible, being coincident with a QRS complex (*circle*), the interval between two manifest waves is twice the basic interval. These small waves are, therefore, sinus P waves: accordingly, A-V dissociation can be diagnosed, revealing a ventricular origin of tachycardia. In diagram (**b**), in contrast, the small positive deflections are arrhythmic: they are not P waves but artifacts

low voltage, since it is relatively easy to detect the small atrial waves whenever these are not "buried" within large QRS or T deflections. This is expressed by the "haystack principle": if you are searching for a needle in a haystack, select a small haystack" (Fig. 6.2).

The bedside diagnosis of A-V dissociation can be improved by heart sound auscultation and arterial pulse palpation: whenever the atrial contraction is dissociated from ventricular activity, it is possible to appreciate a variable loudness of the 1st heart sound and variability in peripheral pulse amplitude. This is because (1) whenever atrial contraction occurs immediately before ventricular systole, the blood flow "opens" the atrioventricular valves, resulting in a relatively loud 1st heart sound, a phenomenon that does not occur if mitral and tricuspid valves are closed at the time of atrial systole, and (2) if atrial contraction occurs when the A-V valves are open, the diastolic ventricular filling is improved, resulting in a relatively increased stroke volume: accordingly, the pulse amplitude will be higher with respect to that of heart beats in which atrial systole occurs while the A-V valves are closed.

6.2.2   Second-Degree V-A Block

In ventricular tachycardia, atrial electrical activity may be not dissociated from ventricular one if retrograde ventricular-atrial (V-A) conduction occurs, as it happens in about one half of cases. The V-A ratio may be 1 (every QRS complex is followed by a

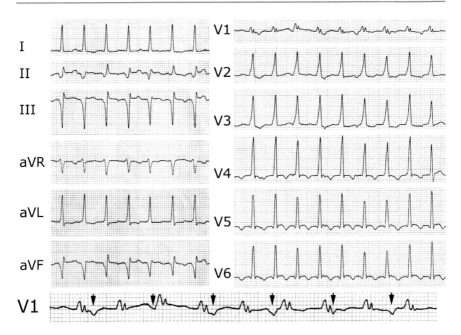

Fig. 6.2 Wide QRS complex tachycardia. QRS duration is 0.12 s, but since in some leads ventricular complexes are relatively narrow, a supraventricular tachycardia could be diagnosed at first glance. The ventricular origin of tachycardia is demonstrated by A-V dissociation; the P waves independent of ventricular complexes (*arrows*), and separated from constant intervals, are easily recognized in lead V1, since in this lead both QRS complexes ant T wave voltages are very low (the haystack principle)

retrograde P wave) or less than 1 when some ventricular impulses are not conducted to the atria. In a wide QRS complex tachycardia, a QRS/P ratio >1 (more QRS complexes than P waves) demonstrates the ventricular origin of the arrhythmia [6–8, 12], (Fig. 6.3), whereas a 1:1 ratio does not permit any definite conclusion since P waves may (a) express a supraventricular tachycardia with 1:1 A-V conduction or (b) represent the retrograde atrial activation during ventricular tachycardia. If analysis of P wave configuration is possible, a main P vector directed inferiorly demonstrates supraventricular origin of the arrhythmia, whereas a P vector directed superiorly (negative P waves in the inferior leads) does not permit any conclusion since not only VT but also several supraventricular tachycardias share a retrograde activation of the atria. In some cases of VT, however, retrograde P waves appear as positive in the inferior leads, a phenomenon that has been called "the illusion of retrograde positive P waves" (Fig. 6.4) [8, 13, 14].

6.2.3   Capture and Fusion Beats

The presence of narrow, or relatively narrow, beats during wide QRS tachycardia suggests a diagnosis of VT, *provided that narrow complexes are preceded by a P wave with an interval consistent with anterograde A-V conduction of the impulse.* The narrow, or less wide, complexes are *capture* or *fusion* beats that occur

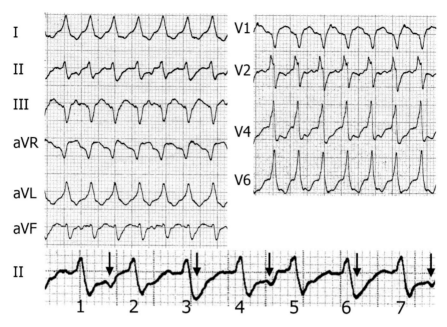

Fig. 6.3 Ventricular tachycardia with 3:2 retrograde block of the Wenckebach type. Lead II (enlarged in the *bottom row*) analysis reveals that ventricular complexes *1, 4,* and *7* are followed by negative P waves occurring midway between two consecutive QRS complexes. Beats *3* and *6,* in turn, show very wide "S waves" that never occur in the other beats, whereas complexes *2* and *5* do not show any of the 2 above characteristics (negative P wave, wide "s wave"). It is, therefore, evident that in a group of 3 beats, the 1st one (complexes *3* and *6*) is followed by a retrograde P wave with a short R-P interval, whereas the P wave following the 2nd beat of the group (complexes *1, 4, 7*) occurs with a relatively long interval, and after the 3rd complex of the series (beats *2* and *5*), no P wave occurs. In other words, there is a retrograde 2nd-degree 3:2 Wenckebach type block, and this establishes the diagnosis of ventricular tachycardia. In this tracing, the r wave peak time in lead II is 30 ms

whenever, during VT, a sinus or supraventricular impulse succeeds in reaching the ventricles, whose depolarization is due totally (capture) or partially (fusion) to that impulse (Fig. 6.5). Capture and fusion beats are reliable signs of VT, but they are rare (4 % in a study based on 96 cases of proved VT [10]) and can be observed only in the presence of A-V dissociation. Since the latter phenomenon is, in itself, a clear sign of VT, the further help provided by capture and fusion beats is trivial, provided that these never occur whenever the heart rate is very high, being the A-V node made always refractory by ectopic ventricular impulses [6, 8].

6.2.4   Precordial QRS Concordance

A "concordant" QRS morphology in all the precordial leads, namely, ventricular complexes totally negative (QS pattern) or positive (R or qR pattern), demon-strates a ventricular origin of tachycardia, since no intraventricular conduction

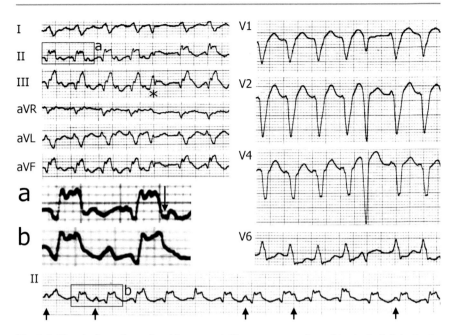

Fig. 6.4 Ventricular tachycardia with retrograde P waves apparently positive in the inferior leads. In all leads, that are simultaneous, apart from the tracing in the bottom strip, the 5th beat (*asterisk*) is a ventricular extrasystole. Beats 1–4 are followed by P waves that seem, at first glance, positive in the inferior leads and negative in aVR and aVL. The premature beat alters the relationship between QRS complexes and P waves, being the last two ventricular beats not followed by P waves. The bottom strip (lead II) has been recorded later with respect to the others and clearly shows A-V dissociation: P waves of sinus origin are positive (*arrows*) and independent of QRS complexes; some sinus P waves, occurring simultaneously with ventricular complexes, are invisible, being "buried" within the ventricular complexes. Panels (**a, b**) show enlarged beats: during retrograde V-A conduction, P waves are negative (*arrow* in section **a**), not positive as they seem at first glance. In section (**b**), a positive P wave is evident in between two QRS complexes, demonstrating A-V dissociation

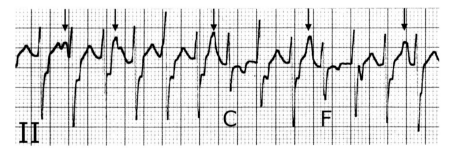

Fig. 6.5 Capture and fusion beats during ventricular tachycardia. In this ECG strip, A-V dissociation is evident (*arrows* point out sinus P waves that modify T wave morphology). In two occasions, the sinus impulse is conducted to the ventricles, giving rise to a narrow QRS complex (capture beat, labeled *C*) or to a fusion beat (labeled *F*). These are intermediate in configuration between ectopic wide complexes and capture beat

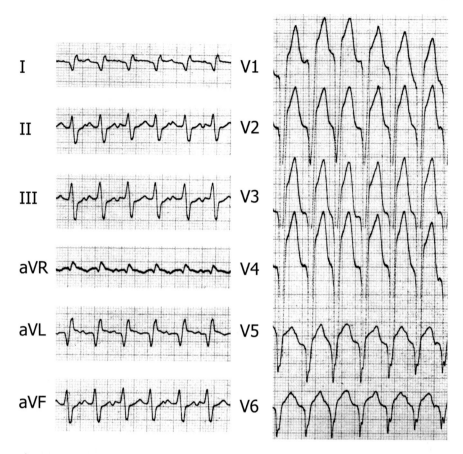

Fig. 6.6 Precordial concordance. In this tachycardia, wide QRS complexes with QS morphology are present in all precordial leads. This pattern demonstrates without any exception the ventricular origin of tachycardia. Analysis of the inferior leads also reveals a 2nd-degree V-A block with 3:2 ratio; the retrograde negative P waves modify the T wave configuration in two consecutive beats, whereas in the 3rd QRS complex, the T wave is not affected

disturbance can result in such a configuration [15]. Concordance, however, cannot be diagnosed if rS, Rs, or rs complexes occur even in one single precordial lead. In a study based on 232 electrocardiograms with bundle branch block analyzed during sinus rhythm, none showed precordial concordance, suggesting a 100 % specificity of this sign indicating the ventricular origin of the arrhythmia [16]. Negative concordance (QS morphology in all precordial leads, Fig. 6.6), however, is specific of VT, whereas positive concordance could be observed, although rarely, in a preexcited tachycardia due to a left-sided Kent bundle [7, 8]. Negative concordance in the bipolar limb leads (I, II, III) has also been proposed as a specific pattern suggesting VT; [17] such a configuration demonstrates an extreme right axis deviation, a phenomenon that never occurs in adults, apart from some cases of congenital heart disease or dextrocardia.

6.2.5 Absence of RS Complexes in the Precordial Leads

In several cases of VT, none of the precordial leads shows ventricular complexes with a configuration characterized by an R wave followed by an S wave (rs, RS, rS, or Rs). This sign, expressing in a slightly different manner the concept of "precordial concordance," suggests a ventricular origin of the arrhythmia. The sign specificity was 100 % both in the original study [5] and in another research based on 133 patients with wide QRS tachycardia; [10] in a different series, however, specificity was 81 and 98 % in the presence of positive and negative precordial QRS complexes, respectively [16].

6.2.6 Interval >100 ms from QRS Complex Beginning to S Wave Nadir in a Precordial Lead

It has been observed that whenever, in a wide QRS complex tachycardia, the interval from QRS complex beginning to S wave nadir exceeds 100 ms in a precordial lead, tachycardia is ventricular in origin [5]. The above criterion was fulfilled in 41 % of patients with previous myocardial infarction and VT [18]. In subjects with slowed down intraventricular conduction, however, leads V4–V6 show at times the above-mentioned sign even during sinus rhythm, particularly in the presence of left axis deviation. In a study based on electrocardiograms with left bundle branch block and sinus rhythm, 34 % of cases had an interval from QRS complex beginning to S wave nadir >100 ms [16], demonstrating a low specificity of this sign in revealing VT.

6.2.7 Vagal Stimulation Maneuvers

In the presence of QRS wide complex tachycardia, vagal stimulation can result in the following responses:

1. No change in tachycardia morphology or rate: the question remains open.
2. Sinus rhythm restoration: supraventricular reentrant tachycardia with a circuit incorporating the A-V node.
3. Variation in A-V conduction ratio, with appearance of P or F waves: atrial tachycardia or atrial flutter.
4. Variation in V-A conduction ratio, demonstrated by QRS complexes not followed by a retrograde P wave: ventricular origin of tachycardia.

6.3 The Electrocardiogram in the Absence of Tachycardia

An ECG recorded in the absence of tachycardia can be at times helpful, since a conduction disturbance or preexcitation observed during sinus rhythm can be the key to recognize the mechanism underlying the wide QRS complexes. In the great majority of cases, however, no ECG recorded during sinus rhythm is available at the moment of the arrhythmic emergence. Whenever the ECG during tachycardia is identical to that obtained in sinus rhythm, the arrhythmia is supraventricular in origin, apart from a single exception: the bundle branch reentry tachycardia [19]. In the latter condition, a tracing in sinus rhythm can be misleading, since it suggests a supraventricular, rather than ventricular, origin of the arrhythmia [19].

6.4   QRS Complex Morphology in Leads V1 and V6

Analysis of QRS complex configuration represents an important tool in wide QRS complex tachycardia. Whenever other diagnostic signs (A-V dissociation, capture and fusion beats, precordial concordance, etc.) are either absent or controversial, the distinction between supraventricular and ventricular tachycardia lies on morphologic analysis of ventricular complexes, taking particularly into account leads V1 and V6. The 1st step is tachycardia classification based on QRS morphology in lead V1: whenever ventricular complex is mainly positive in this lead, tachycardia will be defined as "RBBB type," whereas if in that lead ventricular complexes are negative, tachycardia will be classified as "LBBB type." In any situation, the leads to be analyzed are V1 and V6.

6.4.1   Wide QRS Complex Tachycardia with Right Bundle Branch Block-Type Configuration (Positive QRS Complex in Lead V1)

V1. Ventricular complexes with morphology *R* or *Rr'* (the 1st R wave higher than the 2nd one), as well as *qR* or *RS* complexes, suggest VT, whereas both a triphasic (*rsRÐ* or *rSRÐ*) or biphasic configurations *rRÐ* with the 2nd R wave higher than the 1st one suggest SVT with aberrant conduction (Fig. 6.7).
V6. In this lead, *rS, QS,* or *qR* complexes are specific of VT (Fig. 6.8), whereas *qRs* complexes suggest aberrant conduction (specificity 95 %). Whenever the R/S ratio, however, is <1 (larger S wave than R wave voltage in lead V6), the ventricular, rather than supraventricular, origin of tachycardia is more likely [10, 16, 20].

6.4.2   Wide QRS Complex Tachycardia with Left Bundle Branch Block-Type Morphology (Negative QRS Complex in Lead V1)

V1. In the presence *of SVT with aberrant conduction and LBBB morphology, this lead shows either a QS configuration or a small and relatively narrow (≤30 ms) r wave* followed by a deep S wave with an early (<60 ms) nadir. R wave duration >30 ms or S wave nadir later than 60 ms from the QRS complex beginning suggest ventricular origin of the arrhythmia. Moreover, a notch in the proximal (descending) limb of S wave indicates VT (Fig. 6.8).

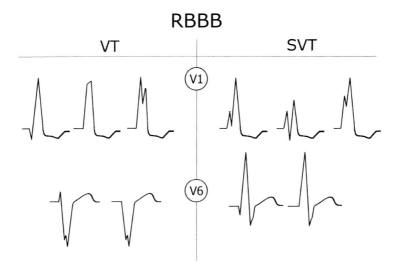

Fig. 6.7 Ventricular complex morphology suggesting either VT or SVT with aberrant conduction in wide QRS complex tachycardia with RBBB-like configuration (QRS complex mainly positive in lead V1)

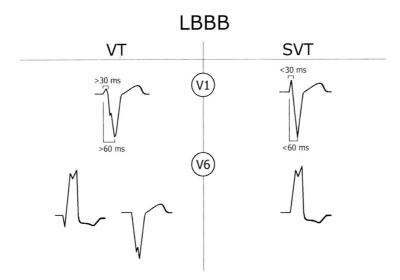

Fig. 6.8 Ventricular complex morphology suggesting either VT or SVT with aberrant conduction in wide QRS complex tachycardia with LBBB-like configuration (QRS complex mainly negative in lead V1)

V6. In a wide QRS complex tachycardia, negative or predominantly *negative QRS complexes in lead V6 suggest at first glance a ventricular origin* of the arrhythmia independent of the associated intraventricular disturbance pattern [20]. Impulses of ventricular origin show often (69 % of cases) a negative net QRS amplitude (algebraic sum of positive and negative deflections) in V6, whereas this pattern is relatively rare (27 % of cases) in supraventricular tachycardia.

These signs based on QRS morphology in leads V1 and V6, introduced by Kindwall [21], express the slow initial progression of the ventricular wave front when the depolarization is not due to an impulse conducted over the His-Purkinje system. In true LBBB, thus, the 1st ventricular vector, expressing the right-to-left septal depolarization, is directed to the left and anteriorly: lead V1, thus, cannot show a *wide* r wave since the initial ventricular depolarization is fast, being the supraventricular impulse conducted over the Purkinje system. Accordingly, *in a broad QRS tachycardia with LBBB configuration, a relatively wide (≥30 ms) r wave in lead V1 strongly suggests a ventricular origin of the arrhythmia.* The same holds true for a relatively late (>60 ms) S wave nadir in lead V1 and for the presence of a notch in the descending S wave limb. The specificity of the above "ectopic" QRS morphologies in lead V1, however, is not 100 %: a study based on electrocardiograms with LBBB during sinus rhythm has reported a specificity of 78, 66 and 66 % for r wave duration in lead V1 >30 ms, S wave nadir >60 ms, and notch in the descending S wave limb, respectively [16].

6.4.3   Limitations of Criteria Based on QRS Morphology in Wide QRS Complex Tachycardia

Despite being useful, morphologic criteria are not absolute; the equations *typical bundle branch block = aberrant conduction, atypical bundle branch block = ventricular tachycardia* suffer some *limitations and may lead to wrong conclusions in patients treated with antiarrhythmic drugs, particularly those belonging to class 1C.* This is because these drugs slow down the intraventricular conduction, resulting in very abnormal ventricular complexes. Patients treated with 1C drugs may show extremely wide QRS complexes during SVT, to the extent that morphological analysis leads to a wrong diagnosis. This occurs not rarely in patients with atrial flutter treated with 1C antiarrhythmic drugs, that result in tachycardia rate reduction, favoring 1:1 A-V conduction of atrial impulses, and QRS complex widening.

6.5   Other Signs

6.5.1   QRS Duration >140 ms

It has been observed that a wide complex tachycardia with QRS duration >0.14 s is very likely ventricular in origin [11], but this criterion has a low specificity, ranging from 43 % [16] to 69 % [10]. Moreover, QRS complexes can be, although rarely, relatively narrow (<0.12 s) in ventricular tachycardia.

6.5.2   QRS Axis Deviation

In several cases of VT, left or right axis deviation occurs [9–11], and rarely the QRS axis is normal (between 0° and +90°) in VT. Superior QRS axis deviation, however, has been considered not suggestive of VT in the presence of ventricular complexes with LBBB configuration, whereas an RBBB morphology is often associated with VT (87 % specificity) [16].

6.5.3   Regularity

Apart from atrial fibrillation and atrial flutter or tachycardia with variable A-V conduction ratio, supraventricular tachycardias are usually regular. This is also true for sustained ventricular tachycardias, although irregularity in itself does not exclude VT, the variability of R-R intervals being not uncommon in focal tachycardias, particularly at the beginning or at the end of tachycardia. Sustained VT cycle variability has also been attributed to exit block [22] or longitudinal dissociation in the reentry pathway of tachycardia [23, 24].

6.6   Lead aVR Analysis

A new algorithm based on lead aVR analysis has recently been proposed to distinguish ectopy from aberrant conduction in wide QRS complex tachycardia [25, 26]. The procedure is based on four steps (Fig. 6.9): the first three ones are simple and quick, whereas the 4th step requires complicated voltage measurements. Whenever the sign looked for in steps 1, 2, or 3 is present, the diagnosis is VT, whereas only in step 4 becomes possible the recognition of SVT with aberrant conduction (Fig. 6.9).

6.6.1   Step 1: Dominant Initial R Wave

146 out of 482 cases of wide QRS tachycardia showed in lead aVR *a dominant initial R wave*, which was the largest ventricular complex deflection (Figs. 6.9 and 6.10). This pattern *demonstrated a ventricular origin* of the arrhythmia, confirmed by intracardiac recordings, in 144/146 cases (sensitivity 38.9 %, specificity 98.2 %).

6.6.2   Step 2: q or r initial Wave with Duration >40 ms
in qR or rS complexes

A ventricular complex starting, in aVR, *not with a dominant R wave but with a low voltage q or r wave whose duration was ≥40 ms* was present in 74 out of 336 cases without a dominant initial R wave. In 65 of these, the diagnosis was VT (sensitivity 28.8 %, specificity 91.8 %).

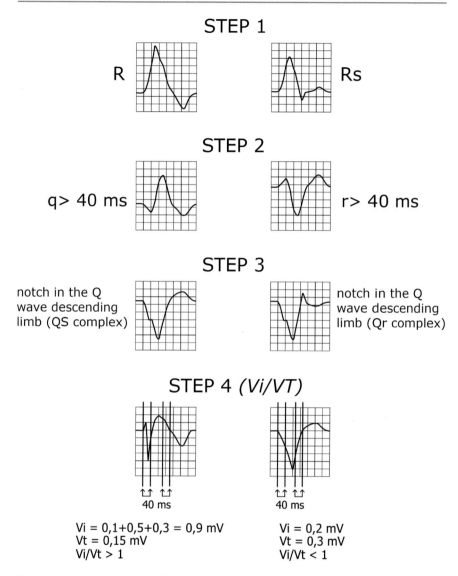

Fig. 6.9 Algorithm based on aVR analysis. *Vi* voltage of the first 40 ms, *Vt* voltage of the final 40 ms (see text)

6.6.3 Step 3: Notch in the Descending Q Wave Limb of a Negative (QS or Qr) Ventricular Complex

This pattern was present in 32 over 37 VT cases where the first 2 criteria were absent (sensitivity 19.9 %, specificity 95 %).

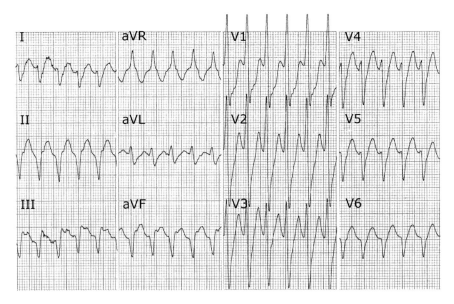

Fig. 6.10 Ventricular tachycardia. In this wide QRS complex tachycardia, negative P waves follow ventricular complexes in the inferior leads. The arrhythmia cannot be classified as "RBBB morphology" or "LBBB morphology" since lead V1 shows complexes with RS configuration. Both QS complexes in lead V6 and aVR analysis (entirely positive complexes) suggest VT

6.6.4   Step 4: *Vi/Vt* Ratio

The presence of any sign in steps 1–3 demonstrates the ventricular origin of the arrhythmia, but *the absence of these criteria does not permit to exclude VT and does not demonstrate SVT.* In this situation it is necessary to evaluate the *Vi/Vt ratio, namely, the ratio between the voltages recorded during the first 40 ms of the QRS complex (Vi) and those measured during the last 40 ms of the complex (Vt).* To calculate *Vi* (initial voltage) and *Vt* (terminal voltage), it is necessary to sum the amplitude of *all the deflections present in the first and the last 40 ms*, respectively (Fig. 6.10). This is not a very easy task, since the authors suggest to measure not the simple voltage of the deflection, but to take into account separately any limb of the waves. For example, if an R wave of 3 mm is present at the beginning of the ventricular complex, the corresponding calculated voltage is 6 mm (3 of the ascending limb + 3 of the descending limb). Unfortunately, it is not easy to distinguish exactly the moment of QRS complex beginning and/or termination, to the extent that the authors suggest to use a simultaneous recording of several leads (at least aVR, aVL, aVF) in order to make easier the identification of QRS complex beginning and/or termination.

A *Vi/Vt ratio ≥1 suggests a diagnosis of SVT* with aberrant conduction, while *a ratio ≤1 speaks in favor of VT.* This criterion has a logical basis: in VT, intraventricular conduction is totally independent of the conduction system, and the ectopic impulse is slowly conducted; accordingly, a small amount of ventricular muscle is

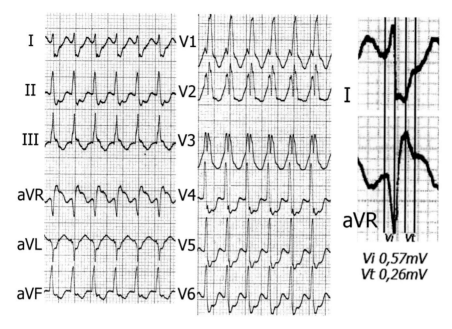

Fig. 6.11 Supraventricular tachycardia with aberrant conduction. Neither P waves nor signs of A-V dissociation are recognizable in this ECG. The morphology of ventricular complexes (rsR′ in V1, Rs with wide s wave in V6) suggests aberrant conduction. The same diagnosis results from lead aVR analysis, since neither dominant initial R wave nor wide q or r wave with duration >40 ms occurs, and is also absent a notch in the proximal q wave limb. Moreover, the ratio between the initial (first 40 ms, *Vi*) and the terminal (final 40 ms, *Vt*) voltage is >1, pinpointing the diagnosis of aberrant conduction

depolarized during the first 40 ms, resulting in a relatively low voltage of the corresponding ECG deflections. When, in contrast, the initial ventricular depolarization occurs using the Purkinje system, as it happens in bundle branch block, a relatively large myocardial mass is depolarized during the first 40 ms, resulting in relatively high voltage-related deflections. Examples of correct diagnosis arrived by means of aVR analysis are reported in Figs. 6.11, 6.12, and 6.13.

In conclusion, aVR analysis can be very helpful whenever one of the signs described in steps 1–3 is present, but becomes less useful in their absence.

6.7   R Wave Peak Time at Lead II

It has recently been reported that the *R wave peak time (RWPT) duration in lead II (the interval from the QRS complex beginning to the 1st change in polarity)* permits a quick and reliable distinction between VT and SVT [27]. The authors have observed that an *RWPT ≤50 ms demonstrates a supraventricular origin* of the arrhythmia, whereas an *RWPT ≥50 ms in lead II suggests VT*. The underlying reason why a long RWPT speaks in favor of ventricular origin of tachycardia is

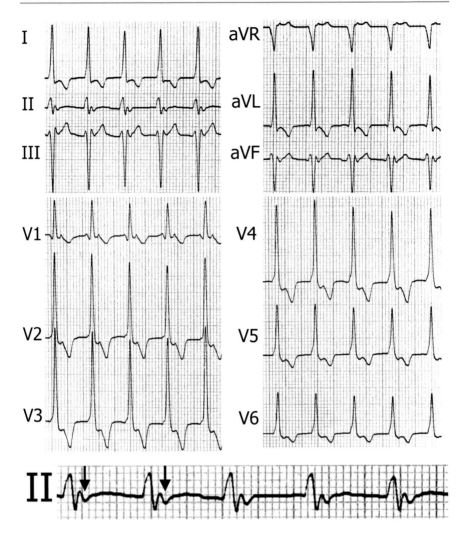

Fig. 6.12 Wide QRS tachycardia with 1:1 V-A conduction. Negative P waves follow ventricular complexes with constant R-P interval in the inferior leads (*arrows* in the *bottom strip*, representing lead II enlarged). This pattern suggests a diagnosis of ventricular (fascicular) tachycardia, despite the relatively narrow QRS complexes

likely the slow initial diffusion of the depolarization wave front in VT. In SVT, in contrast, at the beginning of ventricular depolarization, the supraventricular impulse is normally conducted over a bundle branch (or a fascicle) and the Purkinje system, in such a way that a relatively large myocardial mass is quickly depolarized, resulting in a short RWPT. In the case of VT, in contrast, the cardiac impulse slowly travels over the common myocardial tissue, resulting in a long RWPT. The efficacy of this sign in discriminating VT from SVT is very high in the study that has described such a criterion; the experience of our group,

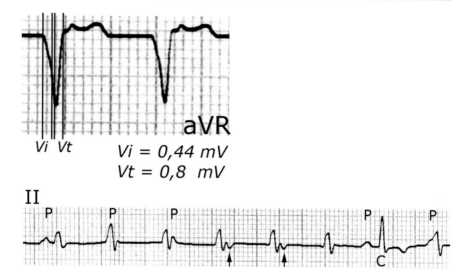

Vi Vt

$Vi = 0,44 \ mV$

$Vt = 0,8 \ mV$

Fig. 6.13 Same case of the preceding figure. Analysis of lead aVR (*top*) and effect of verapamil administration (*bottom*). Despite the absence of (a) dominant initial R wave, (b) q wave with duration >40 ms, (c) notch in the q wave descending limb, the ratio between the voltages of the first and the final 40 ms (*Vi/Vt*) is less than 1, supporting the diagnosis of VT. The ECG recorded during intravenous verapamil administration (strip of lead II) shows A-V dissociation (the 1st three and the last QRS complex) and a capture beat (*C*); *arrows* indicate retrograde conduction restarting

however, is less satisfactory. Further research is necessary to evaluate the real efficacy of RWPT in lead II. Figure 6.3 shows a case of VT in which the RWPT does not exceed 30 ms.

In conclusion, the classic diagnostic criteria to distinguish VT from SVT with aberrant conduction include the following:

1. A-V dissociation, characterized by absence of any relationship between QRS complexes and P waves; this phenomenon is at times immediately recognizable but more often can be discovered only by means of a detailed analysis of the tracing.
2. Second-degree ventriculoatrial block, namely, a relationship between P waves and QRS complexes, but with more ventricular complexes than P waves.
3. Fusion and/or capture beats.
4. Concordant precordial pattern, a sign that can be also expressed as absence of RS (or even rs, Rs, rS) complexes in the precordial leads.
5. Analysis of QRS complexes aimed at discriminating a typical pattern of intraventricular conduction disturbance from a QRS configuration that is impossible or unlikely whenever the ventricular depolarization is dependent on a supraventricular impulse.

Several further criteria have been introduced to identify the origin of wide QRS complex tachycardia, but none of these is able to provide a simple and quick solution of the problem.

Vagal maneuvers and analysis of previous electrocardiograms recorded during sinus rhythm, if available, can provide further keys to the diagnosis. Some criteria proposed in the past, such as QRS axis or ventricular complex duration, are nowadays no longer considered; in addition, it has been demonstrated that items such as age, hemodynamic status, heart rate, and regularity of R-R intervals can be misleading and should not be taken into account.

Analysis of QRS configuration in leads V1 and V6 is a keystone in distinguishing the origin of wide QRS tachycardias: diagnostic criteria rely upon the assumption that aberration is due to a functional bundle branch block, whereas ectopy derives from a totally abnormal activation of the ventricles. Aberration, thus, results in a "typical" bundle branch block morphology, whereas ectopy is expressed by an "atypical" bundle branch block. Specific criteria, based on analysis of leads V1 and V6, have been developed to distinguish from each other the two conditions. Criteria based on QRS configuration, however, suffer from limitations since unexpected complicating factors, such as a previous myocardial infarction, can result in an "atypical" form of bundle branch block even in the presence of supraventricular tachycardia.

Recently proposed items (lead aVR analysis, peak R wave time in lead II) can be at times useful, but they need further investigation to confirm the results obtained by the authors that introduced such criteria.

6.8   Ventricular Versus Preexcited Tachycardia

In preexcited tachycardia, supraventricular impulses are conducted to the ventricles over an accessory pathway, resulting in wide QRS complexes; this is because ventricular depolarization is entirely (or, less commonly, partially) due to the impulse conducted over the abnormal conduction pathway. Such a situation may occur in the presence of (1) atrial tachycardia, (2) atrial flutter, (3) A-V nodal reentrant tachycardia, and (4) antidromic A-V reentrant tachycardia.

In all of these conditions, ventricular depolarization is due to the accessory pathway, and the QRS complexes are very wide ("pure" delta waves), mimicking a VT. It is, thus, necessary to distinguish VT from preexcited tachycardia, since at first glance QRS complex morphology suggests in the latter ventricular, rather than supraventricular, origin of the arrhythmia. In antidromic A-V reentrant tachycardia due to Mahaim fibers, however, the morphology of QRS complexes suggests supraventricular, rather than ventricular, origin of the arrhythmia, since the accessory pathway is usually connected with the right bundle branch, resulting in a typical left bundle branch block pattern [28].

Distinction between VT and preexcited tachycardia is based on the following concept: VT can originate from any part of the ventricular myocardium, whereas in preexcited tachycardia, ventricular depolarization starts (apart the rare exception represented by Mahaim fibers) from the atrioventricular rings, in correspondence of ventricular insertion of the Kent bundle. Accordingly, there is a relatively limited possible patterns, and each of them is characteristic of a defined Kent bundle location. Since the ECG in sinus rhythm permits in most cases a reliable localization of the accessory pathways [29, 30], the question to be raised in the presence of a wide QRS complex tachycardia should be the following: "Is the morphology of this arrhythmia consistent with the typical pattern of ventricular depolarization due to an accessory pathway?" If the answer is "yes," a preexcited tachycardia is possible, whereas in the case of negative answer, such a diagnosis can be excluded.

It has been reported that in a wide QRS complex tachycardia, the following morphologies suggest VT rather than preexcitation: [4]

1. Negative QRS complexes in V4–V6
2. Negative precordial QRS concordance (negative QRS complexes in all precordial leads)
3. Deep Q waves or Qr complexes in a precordial lead except V1

Although Q waves in precordial leads other than V1 are virtually impossible in preexcitation, negative complexes in V4–V6 are not rarely observed in preexcitation due to a posteroseptal accessory pathway, since the superiorly directed vector can result in large S waves.

References

1. Buxton AE, Merchlinsky FE, Daherty JU. Hazards of intravenous Verapamil for sustained ventricular tachycardia. Am J Cardiol. 1987;59:1107–10.
2. Dancy M, Camm AJ, Ward D. Misdiagnosis of chronic recurrent ventricular tachycardia. Lancet. 1985;2:320–3.
3. Stewart RB, Bardy GH, Greene HL. Wide complex tachycardia: misdiagnosis and outcome after emergent therapy. Ann Intern Med. 1986;104:766–71.
4. Antunes E, Brugada J, Steurer G, et al. The differential diagnosis of a regular tachycardia with a wide QRS complex on the 12-lead ECG: ventricular tachycardia, supraventricular tachycardia with aberrant intraventricular conduction, and supraventricular tachycardia with anterograde conduction over an accessory pathway. Pacing Clin Electrophysiol. 1994;17:1515–24.
5. Brugada P, Brugada J, Mont L, et al. A new approach to the differential diagnosis of a regular tachycardia with a wide QRS complex. Circulation. 1991;83:1649–59.
6. Oreto G, Luzza F, Satullo G, et al. Il dilemma del QRS largo. Torino: Centro Scientifico; 1989. p. 17–24.
7. Oreto G, Luzza F, Satullo G, et al. Tachicardia ventricolare: diagnosi all'ECG di superficie. Cardiostimolazione. 1992;11:35–50.
8. Oreto G, Luzza F, Satullo G, et al. I Disordini del Ritmo Cardiaco. Torino: Centro Scientifico; 1997. p. 157–65.
9. Wellens HJJ. Ventricular tachycardia: diagnosis of broad QRS complex tachycardia. Heart. 2001;86:579–85.
10. Drew BJ, Scheinman MM. ECG criteria to distinguish between aberrantly conducted supraventricular tachycardia and ventricular tachycardia: practical aspects for the immediate care setting. Pacing Clin Electrophysiol. 1995;18:2194–208.
11. Wellens HJJ, Bar FWHM, Lie KI. The value of the electrocardiogram in the differential diagnosis of tachycardia with a widened QRS complex. Am J Med. 1978;64:27–33.
12. Schamroth L. I disordini del ritmo cardiaco. Roma: Marrapese; 1980. p. 145–7.
13. Parkin R, Nikolic C, Spodick DH. Upright retrograde P waves during ventricular tachycardia. Am J Cardiol. 1991;68:138–40.

14. Kinoshita S, Okada F. "Upright" retrograde P waves during ventricular tachycardia. Am J Cardiol. 1992;69:711–2.
15. Marriott HJL. Differential diagnosis of supraventricular and ventricular tachycardia. Geriatrics. 1970;25:91–101.
16. Alberca T, Almendral J, Sanz P, et al. Evaluation of the specificity of morphological electro-cardiographic criteria for the differential diagnosis of wide QRS complex tachycardia in patients with intraventricular conduction defects. Circulation. 1997;96:3527–33.
17. Reddy GV, Leghari R. Standard limb lead QRS concordance during wide QRS tachycardia. A new surface ECG sign of ventricular tachycardia. Chest. 1987;92:763–5.
18. Satullo G, Cavalli A, Ferrara MC, et al. Diagnosi elettrocardiografica di tachicardia ventrico-lare in pazienti con pregresso infarto miocardico: frequenza e significato dei diversi criteri diagnostici. G Ital Cardiol. 1991;21:1305–9.
19. Oreto G, Smeets JLRM, Rodriguez LM, et al. Wide complex tachycardia with atrioventricular dissociation and QRS morphology identical to that of sinus rhythm: a manifestation of bundle branch reentry. Heart. 1996;76:541–7.
20. Kremers MS, Wells T, Black W, et al. Differentiation of the origin of wide QRS complex by the net amplitude of QRS in lead V6. Am J Cardiol. 1989;64:1053–6.
21. Kindwall KE, Brown J, Josephson ME. Electrocardiographic criteria for ventricular tachycar-dia in wide complex left bundle branch block morphology tachycardias. Am J Cardiol. 1988;61:1279–83.
22. Oreto G, Luzza F, Satullo G, et al. Non sustained ventricular tachycardia with Wenckebach exit block. J Electrocardiol. 1987;20:51–4.
23. Oreto G, Satullo G, Luzza F, et al. Irregular ventricular tachycardia: a possible manifestation of longitudinal dissociation within the reentry pathways. Am Heart J. 1992;124:1506–11.
24. Satullo G, Oreto G, Donato A, et al. Longitudinal dissociation within the reentry pathway of ventricular tachicardia. Pacing Clin Electrophysiol. 1990;13:1623–8.
25. Vereckei A, Duray G, Szenasi G, et al. Application of a new algorithm in the differential diag-nosis of wide QRS complex tachycardia. Eur Heart J. 2007;28:589–600.
26. Vereckei A, Duray G, Szenasi G, et al. New algorithm using only lead aVR for differential diagnosis of wide QRS complex tachycardia. Heart Rhythm. 2008;5:89–98.
27. Pava LF, Perafan P, Badiel M, et al. R wave peak time at DII: a new criterion for differentiating between wide complex QRS tachycardia. Heart Rhythm. 2010;7:922–6.
28. Bardy GH, Fedor JM, German LD, et al. Surface electrocardiographic clues suggesting pres-ence of a nodofascicular Mahaim fiber. J Am Coll Cardiol. 1984;3:1161–8.
29. Oreto G, Gaita F, Luzza F, et al. L'elettrocardiogramma nella preeccitazione. G Ital Cardiol. 1996;26:303–32.
30. Oreto G, Luzza F, Donato A, et al. L'elettrocardiogramma: un mosaico a 12 tessere. Torino: Centro Scientifico Editore; 2009. p. 223–42.

Acute Management of Arrhythmias in Patients with Known Congenital Heart Disease

7

Francesca Bianchi and Stefano Grossi

7.1 Focusing on the Issue

Surgical advances for congenital heart disease (CHD) allow long-term survival for a unique group of patients who would otherwise have died during early childhood. Improved longevity had eventually exposed to late complications, atrial and ventricular arrhythmias contributing to sudden cardiac death (SCD) [1]. Arrhythmias are the consequences of both native abnormalities and surgical procedures. It seems that the arrhythmic burden is the price paid to survival and mostly occurs in adults with CHD. It is now estimated that there are over 1.8 million of adult patients with CHD in Europe [2] and one million in North America [1].

Some defects are best known since studies have focused on specific lesions with predilection for common malformations with effective surgical solution and large number of patients surviving into middle age: this is the case of tetralogy of Fallot that has been studied more extensively than other conditions and so arrhythmic mechanisms and risks are best known [1]; other conditions, less common or with a more recent improvement of survival, are less known.

The entire spectrum of arrhythmias may be encountered in adults with CHD, with several subtypes often coexisting. For some conditions, arrhythmias are intrinsic to the structural malformation itself, as is the case with Wolff-Parkinson-White syndrome in the setting of Ebstein's anomaly, twin atrioventricular (AV) node tachycardia in heterotaxy, or AV block in the setting of "congenitally corrected" transposition of the great arteries (L-TGA). For most other CHD patients, arrhythmias represent an acquired condition related to the unique myocardial substrate

F. Bianchi (✉) • S. Grossi
Cardiology Unit, Department of Cardiovascular Diseases, Azienda Ospedaliera Ordine Mauriziano, Turin, Italy
e-mail: fbianchi@mauriziano.it; sgrossi@mauriziano.it

© Springer International Publishing Switzerland 2016
M. Zecchin, G. Sinagra (eds.), *The Arrhythmic Patient in the Emergency Department: A Practical Guide for Cardiologists and Emergency Physicians*, DOI 10.1007/978-3-319-24328-3_7

created by surgical scars in conjunction with cyanosis and abnormal pressure/volume loads of long duration [3, 4].

Arrhythmia substrate and consequent management is peculiar for any CHD, but some general principles can be identified, and recently international scientific boards have provided evidence-based recommendations on best practice procedures for the evaluation, diagnosis, and management of arrhythmias [5, 6].

Arrhythmia management is strictly connected to anatomical native and surgical substrate and to hemodynamic status. Classification of CHD complexity (simple, moderate, and great/severe) proposed by the ACC/AHA task force [7] reported in Table 7.1 is used to orientate management.

7.2   What Physicians Working in ED Should Know

Facing acute arrhythmias in CHD patients needs an early interplay between emergency physician and cardiologists.

Hemodynamically poorly tolerated tachycardia or ventricular fibrillation resulting in pulseless arrest requires management according to AHA/ACC/ESC guidelines for Adult Cardiac Life Support (ACLS) [8]. When direct current cardioversion is required, paddles or patches have to be positioned taking into account cardiac location in the chest [6].

In tolerated arrhythmias, 12-lead electrocardiogram (ECG) of the event should be registered. Knowledge of anatomical defect and collection of surgical reports are also fundamental for best acute and long-term management and should be obtained as soon as possible.

Hemodynamically tolerated tachycardia should be managed according to well-established adult guidelines, while taking into consideration CHD-specific issues [6] on drug therapy: antiarrhythmic drugs (AAD) are frequently poorly tolerated due to negative inotropic and other side effects, and few data exist on their safety and efficacy [6].

For atrial arrhythmias the *thromboembolic risk* must be assessed before cardioversion, reminding that in moderate and severe complexity CHD, it is high even when onset is <48 h [6].

Unexplained syncope in adults with CHD is an alarming event that may have several potential etiologies, including conduction abnormalities and bradyarrhythmias, atrial and/or ventricular arrhythmias, and nonarrhythmic causes [6].

In patients with CHD, the majority of *sudden cardiac deaths* (SCD) have an arrhythmic etiology, but up to 20 % may be nonarrhythmic, as in cerebral or pulmonary embolism, myocardial infarction, heart failure, and aortic or aneurysmal rupture [5]. SCD is responsible for approximately one-fifth of the mortality in adult's CHD, with a greater risk observed in certain malformations (tetralogy of Fallot, Ebstein's disease, left-sided obstructive disease). However, the annual mortality rates are low compared with adult population (0.1–0.3 % per patient-year) [1].

Table 7.1 Complexity of diagnosis in adult patients with congenital heart disease

Simple	Moderate complexity	Great/severe complexity

Native disease:
Isolated congenital aortic valve disease
Isolated congenital mitral valve disease (except parachute valve, cleft leaflet)
Small atrial septal defect
Isolated small ventricular septal defect (no associated lesions)
Mild pulmonary stenosis
Small patent ductus arteriosus
Repaired conditions:
Previously ligated or occluded ductus arteriosus
Repaired secundum or sinus venosus atrial septal defect without residua
Repaired ventricular septal defect without residua
	Aorto-left ventricular fistulas
	Anomalous pulmonary venous drainage, partial or total
	Atrioventricular septal defects, partial or complete
	Coarctation of the aorta
	Ebstein's anomaly
	Infundibular right ventricular outflow obstruction of significance
	Ostium primum atrial septal defect
	Patent ductus arteriosus (not closed)
	Pulmonary valve regurgitation, moderate to severe
	Pulmonary valve stenosis, moderate to severe
	Sinus of Valsalva fistula/aneurysm
	Sinus venosus atrial septal defect Subvalvular or supravalvular aortic stenosis
	Tetralogy of Fallot
	Ventricular septal defect with:
	    Absent valve or valves
	    Aortic regurgitation
	Coarctation of the aorta
	  Mitral disease
	  Right ventricular outflow tract obstruction
	  Straddling tricuspid or mitral valve
	  Subaortic stenosis
		Conduits, valved or nonvalved
		Cyanotic congenital heart disease (all forms)
		Double-outlet ventricle
		Eisenmenger syndrome
		Fontan procedure
		Mitral atresia
		Single ventricle (also called double inlet or outlet, common, or primitive)
		Pulmonary atresia (all forms)
		Pulmonary vascular obstructive disease
		Transposition of the great arteries
		Tricuspid atresia
		Truncus arteriosus/hemitruncus
		Other abnormalities of atrioventricular or ventriculoarterial connection not included above (e.g., crisscross heart, isomerism, heterotaxy syndromes, ventricular inversion)

Adapted from Warnes et al. [7]; with permission

7.3   What Cardiologist Should Know

Atrial tachyarrhythmias (ATs), the most frequent in CHD, have been identified as a risk factor for SCD. The mechanism has been attributed to rapid AV conduction, most notably at times of exertion, with hemodynamic instability caused by the atrial tachyarrhythmia itself or by its degeneration into a secondary ventricular tachyarrhythmia [7].

Prevalence of ATs is 3 times higher than what is observed in general population, and it is reported that 20-year-old patients with CHD have an equivalent risk of a 55-year-old women without CHD: patients with CHD are young with aged hearts [9]; atrial fibrillation (AF) is less common than atrial flutter accounting for 20–30 % of all ATs [10, 11].

The most common mechanism of tachycardia seen in the adult CHD patient population is macro-reentry within the atrial muscle. It is defined as *intra-atrial reentrant tachycardia (IART)* [7].

This arrhythmia usually is a late postoperative disorder, and it may arise after nearly all procedures involving a right atriotomy (even simple closure of an atrial septal defect); the incidence is clearly highest after the Mustard–Senning and Fontan operations, in which 30–50 % can be expected to develop a symptomatic episode during follow-up. Generally, IART tends to be slower than typical flutter, with atrial rates in the range of 170–250 beats per minute. In the setting of a healthy AV node, these rates will frequently allow a pattern of 1:1 AV conduction that may result in hemodynamic instability, syncope, or possibly death [3, 7]. Rate control should be achieved as soon as possible. Beta-blocking drugs and nondihydropyridine calcium channel antagonists can be used to achieve ventricular rate control with insufficient evidence to recommend one agent over another; since beta-blockers are associated with a decreased incidence of ventricular tachyarrhythmias in many conditions, it may be reasonable to liberalize their use in this patient population if well tolerated [6].

Sustained IART or AF lasting ≥48 h is an established *risk for thromboembolism* [12, 13], but moderate and complex forms of CHD have a predisposition to thromboembolic complications estimated to be10- to100-fold higher than in age-matched controls: in these patients it may be prudent to rule out intracardiac thrombus prior to cardioversion regardless of the duration of IART or AF [6].

Once atrial arrhythmia is recognized and thromboembolic risk ruled out, acute interruption can be performed with electrical cardioversion, overdrive pacing (in patients with implanted atrial or dual chamber pacemaker/defibrillators), or antiarrhythmic drugs.

Reciprocating tachycardia and some non-automatic focal atrial tachycardias may be terminated by vagal maneuvers, intravenous adenosine, or non-dihydropyridine calcium channel antagonists, with the exception of patients with an anterograde conducting accessory pathway (WPW).

There is a paucity of literature regarding pharmacologic conversion of IART or AF in adults with CHD; ibutilide has been tested in a small pediatric series [14], but there are no efficacy and safety data regarding acute conversion of IART or atrial fibrillation with class IA and IC and other class III drugs in patients with CHD [6]: *electrical cardioversion should therefore be preferred.* Anterior–posterior pad positioning may be needed in the setting of marked atrial dilation [5].

Experience with chronic pharmacologic therapy for IART in adults with CHD has been discouraging [6, 10, 11, 15], resulting in a growing preference for non-pharmacologic options in most centers.

Nevertheless, in those with moderate or complex forms of CHD, a rhythm control treatment strategy (i.e., maintenance of sinus rhythm) is generally preferred to rate control as the initial management approach [6].

Ventricular arrhythmias. There are several scenarios in which high-grade ventricular arrhythmias may develop in CHD. The most familiar involves macroreentrant VT as a late complication in postoperative patients who have undergone ventriculotomy and/or patching such as tetralogy of Fallot repair which is the best studied. Reentry circuit is caused by conduction corridors around regions of scar in the RV outflow tract (RVOT). The incidence of late VT or SCD for repaired tetralogy has been estimated between 0.5 and 6.0 % in various series [3, 7]. Some patients with slow organized VT may be hemodynamically stable at presentation, but VT tends to be rapid for the majority, producing syncope or cardiac arrest as the presenting symptom. Serious ventricular arrhythmias may also develop in a number of other malformations, even in the absence of direct surgical scarring to ventricular muscle when the right ventricle supports the systemic circulation or in the presence of a failing systemic ventricle. The appearance of ventricular arrhythmias in these cases commonly coincides with deterioration in hemodynamic status [7].

Cardioversion should be expeditiously performed for any sustained ventricular arrhythmia; electrical cardioversion in tolerated arrhythmias has the disadvantage of requiring sedation, while drugs carry the disadvantage of delayed effect.

The most efficacious pharmacologic agent is intravenous amiodarone; this agent may be associated with hypotension if administered rapidly: patients should be continuously observed and intravenous sedation and cardioversion readily available. Beta-blockers can be combined to amiodarone to improve rhythm stability, while lidocaine is a third-choice drug for short-term treatment [8].

When triggered activity is the suspected underlying mechanism, intravenous beta-blockers or calcium channel antagonists may be used, but the latter can be more harmful in the presence of scar-related macroreentry or ischemic ventricular tachycardia [6, 8].

7.4 Indications for Hospitalization, Follow-Up, and Referral

Guidelines recommend that health care for adults with CHD and arrhythmias should be coordinated by regional adult CHD centers of excellence with multidisciplinary staff that serve the surrounding medical community for consultation and referral [5–7, 16].

Syncope, ventricular arrhythmias, and in general arrhythmias in the setting of moderate to severe complexity CHD should be hospitalized.

The onset of arrhythmias may be a signal of hemodynamic decompensation, and the risk associates may be amplified in the presence of the abnormal underlying circulation [16]; a new evaluation with echocardiography and eventually further imaging (transesophageal echocardiogram, MRI/CT scan) or catheterization should be planned after a new-onset arrhythmic event.

Unexplained syncope and "high-risk" CHD substrates should be evaluated with an *electrophysiologic study,* which is also useful in life-threatening arrhythmias or resuscitated sudden cardiac death when the proximate cause for the event is unknown or there is potential for ablation [5, 6].

Before planning any invasive procedure, patients should undergo an individualized and multidisciplinary evaluation and the best knowledge of cardiac and vascular anatomy achieved [5, 6].

Patients with *AF/flutter/IART* and simple forms of CHD could be reasonably managed according to AF guidelines for AF or flutter and no or minimally heart disease [6, 12, 13] for rate/rhythm control strategies as well for anticoagulation: in *nonvalvular simple CHD,* CHADSVASC and HASBLD score should be used and either vitamin K antagonists (VKA) or a novel anticoagulant (NOAC) can be used [5].

In all patients initial therapy for atrial arrhythmias should include adequate rate control, best performed with beta-blockers, if tolerated.

Late postoperative atrial tachyarrhythmias in adults with CHD are most often due to *cavotricuspid isthmus-dependent,* and catheter ablation has proven to be safe and considerably effective, generally preferred over long-term pharmacologic management [6].

In CHD of moderate to severe complexity, an initial strategy of rhythm control is reasonable [5], and patients should be treated with VKA; NOAC is not recommended in this context due to lack of safety data [5, 6]. Non-pharmacologic strategy for rhythm control should be preferred to long-term pharmacologic therapy even if acute success rates of catheter ablation (CA) in CHD seem to be lower compared with the general adult population [5, 11]. If catheter ablation is not feasible or unsuccessful, long-term pharmacologic therapy can be necessary [6, 7]. Class I drugs and dronedarone are not recommended in this setting. *Sotalol* can be considered in patients with preserved ventricular function and without renal insufficiency, hypokalemia, severe sinus node dysfunction, or QT prolongation; *amiodarone* can be considered as first-line antiarrhythmic agent for the long-term maintenance of sinus rhythm in the presence of pathologic hypertrophy of the systemic ventricle, systemic or subpulmonary ventricular dysfunction, or coronary artery disease; in all other conditions, it is a second-line therapy due to high time and dose-dependent side effects; induced thyrotoxicosis is especially common in women with CHD and cyanotic heart disease or univentricular hearts with Fontan palliation and in those with a body mass index $\leq$21 kg/m2 [5, 14]. *Dofetilide* appears to be a reasonable alternative to amiodarone in normal QT patients if available [5].

Rate control may be the definitive therapeutic strategy after failed attempts at rhythm control and in whom rate control is well tolerated [6].

Catheter ablation is also recommended in recurrent symptomatic and/or drug-refractory supraventricular tachycardia related to accessory AV connections or twin AV nodes and in high-risk or multiple accessory pathways and can be beneficial for recurrent symptomatic and/or drug-refractory AV nodal reentrant tachycardia [5, 6].

Ventricular arrhythmias: ICD is the first-line therapy for the secondary prevention of sudden death in adults with CHD [17] and should be considered in high-risk patients [5, 6, 8, 15, 19].

Abnormal systemic venous pathways, impaired or lack of venous access to the ventricle, or right-sided AV valve disease may need *epicardial and/or subcutaneous coils* [5].

The subcutaneous ICD may be a reasonable option in adults with CHD in whom transvenous access is not possible or desirable and in whom anti-bradycardia and ATP functions are not essential [5].

Beta-blockers are associated with a decreased incidence of ventricular tachyarrhythmias in patients with transposition of the great arteries and atrial switch surgery, and they should be used in long-term VA prevention if tolerated [5, 6].

Catheter ablation is indicated as adjunctive therapy to an ICD in adults with CHD and recurrent monomorphic ventricular tachycardia, a ventricular tachycardia storm, or multiple appropriate shocks that are not manageable by device reprogramming or drug therapy [6]. The most common CHD associated with sustained ventricular tachycardia is tetralogy of Fallot: a macroreentry mechanism is at the base of monomorphic ventricular tachycardias, which can be cured with catheter ablation as an alternative to drug therapy; in limited Fallot series after VT ablation, ICD was considered necessary only if CA was unsuccessful [16, 18].

Frequent ventricular ectopy associated with deteriorating ventricular function can reasonably be treated by catheter ablation.

References

1. Walsh EP. Sudden death in adult congenital heart disease: risk stratification in 2014. Heart Rhythm. 2014;11(10):1735–42.
2. Moons P, et al. Delivery of care for adult patients with congenital heart disease in Europe: results from the Euro Heart Survey. Eur Heart J. 2006;27:1324–30.
3. Mondésert B, Dubin AM, Khairy P. Diagnostic tools for arrhythmia detection in adults with congenital heart disease and heart failure. Heart Fail Clin. 2014;10(1):57–67.
4. Walsh EP, Cecchin F. Arrhythmias in adult patients with congenital heart disease. Circulation. 2007;115:534–45.
5. Khairy P, Van Hare GF, Balaji S, Berul CI, Cecchin F, Cohen MI, et al. PACES/HRS expert consensus statement on the recognition and management of arrhythmias in adult congenital heart disease: developed in partnership between the pediatric and congenital electrophysiology society (PACES) and the heart rhythm society (HRS). endorsed by the governing bodies of PACES, HRS, the american college of cardiology (ACC), the american heart association (AHA), the european heart rhythm association (EHRA), the canadian heart rhythm society (CHRS), and the international society for adult congenital heart disease (ISACHD). Can J Cardiol. 2014;30(10):e1–63.
6. Khairy P, Van Hare GF, Balaji S, et al. PACES/HRS expert consensus statement on the recognition and management of arrhythmias in adult congenital heart disease: Developed in partnership between the pediatric and congenital electrophysiology society (PACES) and the heart rhythm society (HRS). endorsed by the governing bodies of PACES, HRS, the american college of cardiology (ACC), the american heart association (AHA), the european heart rhythm association (EHRA), the canadian heart rhythm society (CHRS), and the international society for adult congenital heart disease (ISACHD). Heart Rhythm. 2014;11(10):e102–65.
7. Warnes CA, Williams RG, Bashore TM, et al. ACC/AHA 2008 guidelines for the management of adults with congenital heart disease: A report of the american college of Cardiology/American heart association task force on practice guidelines (writing committee to develop guidelines on the management of adults with congenital heart disease) developed I n collabora-

tion with the american society of echocardiography, heart rhythm society, international society for adult congenital heart disease, society for cardiovascular angiography and interventions, and society of thoracic surgeons. J Am Coll Cardiol. 2008;52(23):e143–26.

8. Pedersen CT, Kay GN, Kalman J, et al. EHRA/HRS/APHRS expert consensus on ventricular arrhythmias. Heart Rhythm. 2014;11(10):e166–96.

9. Bouchardy J, Therrien J, Pilote L, et al. Atrial arrhythmias in adults with congenital heart disease. Circulation. 2009;120:1679–86.

10. Lafuente-Lafuente C, Longas-Tejero MA, Bergmann JF, Belmin J. Antiarrhythmics for maintaining sinus rhythm after cardioversion of atrial fibrillation. Cochrane Database Syst Rev. 2012;5, CD005049.

11. Koyak Z, Kroon B, de Groot JR, et al. Efficacy of antiarrhythmic drugs in adults with congenital heart disease and supraventricular tachycardias. Am J Cardiol. 2013;112:1461e1467.

12. Anderson JL, Halperin JL, Albert NM, et al. Management of patients with atrial fibrillation:a report of the American College of Cardiology/American Heart Association Task Force on Practice Guidelines. J Am Coll Cardiol. 2013;61:1935–44.

13. January CT, Wann LS, Alpert JS, et al. AHA/ACC/HRS guideline for the management of patients with atrial fibrillation. Circulation. 2014;130(23):2071–104.

14. Hoyer AW, Balaji S. The safety and efficacy of ibutilide in children and in patients with congenital heart disease. Pacing Clin Electrophysiol. 2007;30:1003–8.

15. Thorne SA, Barnes I, Cullinan P, Somerville J. Amiodarone-associated thyroid dysfunction: risk factors in adults with congenital heart disease. Circulation. 1999;100(2):149–54.

16. Baumgartner H, Bonhoeffer P, De Groot N, et al. ESC Guidelines for the management of grown-up congenital heart disease (new version 2010) The Task Force on the Management of Grown-up Congenital Heart Disease of the European Society of Cardiology (ESC) Endorsed by the Association for European Paediatric Cardiology (AEPC). Eur Heart J. 2010;31:2915.

17. Zipes DP, Camm AJ, Borggrefe M, et al. ACC/AHA/ESC 2006 guidelines for management of patients with ventricular arrhythmias and the prevention of sudden cardiac death. J Am Coll Cardiol. 2006;48:e247–346.

18. Furushima H, Chinushi M, Sugiura H, et al. Ventricular tachycardia late after repair of congenital heart disease: efficacy of combination therapy with radiofrequency catheter ablation and class III antiarrhythmic agents and long-term outcome. J Electrocardiol. 2006;39:219–24.

19. Priori SG, Blomstrom-Lundqvist C, Mazzanti A, et al. 2015 ESC Guidelines for the management of patients with ventricular arrhythmias and the prevention of sudden cardiac death. Eur Heart J 2015 PMID 26320108.

Acute Management of Arrhythmias in Patients with Channelopathies

8

Francesca Bianchi and Stefano Grossi

The term "channelopathies" defines a group of inherited arrhythmic syndromes caused by mutations of genes encoding for proteins that regulate ion currents [1] in patients without structural heart disease. Mutations disrupt the balance in the cardiac action potential favoring peculiar ECG abnormalities and the risk of life-threatening arrhythmias.

A gain or a loss of function of ionic channels or trafficking proteins underlies the development of arrhythmogenic triggers and substrate and the amplification of transmural heterogeneities [2]. It is estimated that inherited arrhythmia disorders (long and short QT syndrome, Brugada syndrome, catecholaminergic polymorphic ventricular tachycardia, early repolarization syndrome, idiopathic ventricular fibrillation) cause 10 % of the 1.1 million sudden deaths in Europe and the USA [3].

Due to the peculiarity of these rare disorders, some of the commonly used emergency protocols should be applied with caution, since some of antiarrhythmic and resuscitation drugs could be contraindicated and potentially worsen arrhythmias in this specific group of patients.

The congenital *long QT syndromes (LQTS)* are the most common channelopathies, with an estimated prevalence of 1:2000–2500 [4], and are characterized by prolonged repolarization, resulting in a prolonged QT interval on the ECG, and by a susceptibility to polymorphic ventricular arrhythmias known as torsades de pointes [2]. Causes for this primary electrical myocardial disease are mutations in genes coding for cardiac potassium and sodium channels and proteins associating with potassium channels, or mutations in the ankyrin-B gene, that reduce net repolarization currents in the ventricular myocardium prolonging repolarization phase and predispose to early afterdepolarization (EAD)-induced triggered activity. Once

F. Bianchi (✉) • S. Grossi
Cardiology Unit, Department of Cardiovascular Diseases, Azienda Ospedaliera Ordine Mauriziano, Turin, Italy
e-mail: fbianchi@mauriziano.it

© Springer International Publishing Switzerland 2016
M. Zecchin, G. Sinagra (eds.), *The Arrhythmic Patient in the Emergency Department: A Practical Guide for Cardiologists and Emergency Physicians,*
DOI 10.1007/978-3-319-24328-3_8

triggered by EADs, torsades de pointes can be maintained by a reentrant mechanism [1, 4–6].

Short QT syndrome (SQTS), characterized by a short QT interval on ECG with a high sharp T wave and a reduced repolarization phase, has a high familial incidence of palpitations, atrial fibrillation, syncope, and SCD [7, 8], typically during childhood. It is considered the most lethal channelopathy; incidence and prevalence are difficult to determine due to limited data [4, 6–8].

The *Brugada syndrome (BrS)* is an autosomal dominant inherited arrhythmic disorder characterized by an ECG pattern consisting in coved-type ST segment elevation in atypical right bundle branch block in right precordial leads (V1–V3) and risk of SCD resulting from episodes or polymorphic ventricular arrhythmias [9–11]; men are affected with a ratio 8:1 in respect to women; reported prevalence in Europe is 1:2000, while in Asian population, it is 2,4:2000; life-threatening events typically involve young male adults (30–40 years old) during sleep [6, 11].

Catecholaminergic polymorphic ventricular tachycardia (CPVT) is a rare but highly malignant genetic disease leading to an increase in intracellular Ca^{++} concentration, resulting in polymorphic arrhythmias due to a cascade of delayed afterdepolarization and triggered activity occurring during emotional or physical stress that cause syncope and high mortality (30 % by the age of 30 years); the estimated prevalence is 1:10,000 [4, 12].

Recently, several studies have reported that J-point and ST segment elevation in the inferior or lateral leads, which is also called early repolarization (ER) pattern, can be associated with ventricular fibrillation (VF) and SCD in patients without apparent structural heart diseases. However, J-wave elevation is fairly commonly seen in young healthy individuals (estimated prevalence, 1–9 %) and frequently considered to be benign [6]: the vast majority of patients with the ECG pattern are asymptomatic and have a low arrhythmic risk, while strategies for risk stratification remain suboptimal. It is reported that unexplained syncope in patients with an ER pattern, particularly with a "malignant variant" of the pattern, may be an important predictor of future arrhythmic events [4, 13]; the presence of an ER pattern with otherwise unexplained ventricular arrhythmia is commonly referred to as *ER syndrome* [4, 6, 13, 14].

8.1   Focusing on the Issue

The ED physician could deal with a patient with an already established diagnosis of inherited arrhythmia, eventually already treated with drugs and or implanted cardiac defibrillator (ICD).

On the other hand, the referral event could be the first clinical manifestation of an unrecognized inherited arrhythmogenic disorder that, especially in young and otherwise healthy subject, must be suspected, investigated, and finally confirmed or ruled out.

All patients with a known or suspected channelopathy who refer for arrhythmic suggestive symptoms should be ECG monitored and a cardiologic evaluation sought.

Patients resuscitated from cardiac arrest must be rapidly evaluated for the presence of structural heart disease, an inherited arrhythmia syndrome, a triggering ventricular arrhythmia focus, or a noncardiac cause [15].

Most of inherited arrhythmic disorders could be diagnosed on the basis of a standard 12-lead ECG that should therefore be obtained as soon as possible as the chance to make a correct diagnosis is highest in proximity of the arrhythmic event [15]. This is a simple and useful instrument to confirm the presence or suspect a channelopathy, aside from excluding other acquired acute cardiac conditions (such as acute coronary syndrome); however, a single normal resting ECG may not exclude all forms of channelopathies. ECG recording of arrhythmic event, when possible, could be useful for the subsequent management [15].

In all cases it is indicated to avoid pro-arrhythmic triggering conditions and discontinue potentially harmful drugs that are specific for any different channelopathy: currently used antiarrhythmic and resuscitation drugs may hasten the electrical instability in these particular patients and should be therefore avoided when a specific channelopathy is known or suspected (see below).

8.2 Different Ways of Presentation

Cardiac arrest and hemodynamic nontolerated arrhythmias should be managed with early defibrillation [15] with special considerations required for drug administration.

Polymorphic ventricular tachycardia is defined as ventricular rhythm faster than 100 bpm with clearly defined QRS complexes that change continuously from beat to beat; it is the typical life-threatening arrhythmia observed in patients with channelopathies; its occurrence, in the absence of structural heart disease, suggests the presence of an inherited arrhythmia syndrome [15]; it could be self-terminating or degenerate into VF.

Bidirectional ventricular tachycardia, characterized by two alternating QRS complex morphologies with different polarity, is recognized as a hallmark of CPVT; it can degenerate into polymorphic ventricular tachycardia and VF. It may be encountered also in the rarest Andersen-Tawil syndrome and in several other conditions which predispose to delayed afterdepolarizations (DADs) and triggered activity (i.e., digitalis intoxication) [4, 16] See Fig. 8.2.

The term *torsades de pointes* (TdP) was coined by Dessertenne [17] in 1966 as a polymorphic ventricular tachycardia characterized by a pattern where the QRS complexes appear to be twisting around the isoelectric baseline [15]. The trigger for TdP is thought to be a PVC that results from an EAD generated during the abnormally prolonged repolarization phase; this arrhythmia has a typical long-short ventricular cycle length as initiating sequence and is typical for congenital or acquired long QT syndrome. TdP usually self-terminates and it is often responsible for syncopal episodes but when it deteriorates into VF may cause sudden death [4] see fig. 8.2. Since TdP is strongly associated with drugs or electrolyte imbalances that further delay repolarization, precipitating factors should promptly be searched and corrected [15, 18, 19].

Ventricular tachycardia/ventricular fibrillation storm represents a true medical emergency that requires a multidisciplinary approach to care [15] (see Chap. 11).

In patients with known diagnosis of channelopathy (including known gene carriers), the occurrence of *syncope* is an independent predictor of life-threatening arrhythmic events [4].

In most patients, syncope is the first clinical manifestation of inherited arrhythmic disorders that should therefore be evaluated.

Atrial fibrillation (AF) affects 1–2 % of the population and increases in prevalence with aging [20]. Ion channel disorders can predispose to atrial fibrillation, and prevalence in this population is increased, since the same imbalance of the action potential that causes ventricular arrhythmias could affect the atria. On the contrary, AF could be the first manifestation of an inherited cardiac arrhythmia (sometimes unmasked by drug administration [21]) which should be always considered in young otherwise healthy subjects.

Since commonly used drugs for rhythm or heart rate control may be contraindicated due to the potentially life-threatening pro-arrhythmic effect, a non-pharmacological strategy should be considered, with immediate electrical cardioversion always indicated in poorly tolerated AF, but also drugs for anesthesia/sedation should carefully be considered as potentially harmful: for example, propofol should be avoided in Brugada patients, who have a reported prevalence of atrial fibrillation between 9 to 25 and 39 % [21]. Short QT syndrome is characterized by atrial fibrillation [7, 8] with young age onset, being the first clinical manifestation in several reported SQTS cases, since a short repolarization time is a known mechanism in AF [22]: it was observed in 15 % of SQTS population, also younger than 35 years [23]. Adrenergically mediated atrial arrhythmias are also common manifestation of CPVT [4]. In LQTS frequent short-lasting atrial arrhythmias have been reported [23, 24].

Patients presenting with *ICD discharge* should be ECG monitored and device interrogation, even by remote monitoring when available, performed as soon as possible: appropriate shocks due to ventricular arrhythmia should be promptly managed, according to the peculiar diagnosis of the patient. Inappropriate shocks (which may have a high incidence in this population due to young age, high incidence of AF, and sometimes peculiar ECG [25] leading to incorrect recognition of the rhythm) and discharges on non-sustained VT should be avoided as part of the emergency treatment: painful shocks can increase the sympathetic tone and trigger further arrhythmias leading to a malignant cycle of ICD shocks and even death [15]; inhibition through magnet application could be the first intervention before device specialist intervention in case of incessant and clearly inappropriate shocks.

Therapy: The first step of management of acute events in these patients is to avoid and correct potentially triggering conditions:

Fever: In *Brugada* syndrome avoidance of fever is generally accepted to be an important part of prophylactic treatment since it is a well-known trigger of cardiac events [26, 45, 27]. Fever can also be a risk factor for the development of life-threatening ventricular arrhythmias in the *LQT2* form of congenital long QT syndrome [28, 29].

Autonomic influences play an important role in unmasking the electrocardio-graphic phenotype and precipitating lethal arrhythmias. Sympathetic stimulation precipitates tachyarrhythmias and sudden cardiac death in CPVT and LQTS, while in BrS and ER, it can prevent them [30]. Most episodes of VF in patients with Brugada syndrome and some in LQT3 are observed during periods of high vagal tone, such as at rest, during sleep, or after alcohol intake [30]. In LQTS 1 and 2 and CPVT patients, sympathetic stimulation and sympathomimetic drugs should be avoided, and the use of sedation to reduce emotional stress may be considered as a support to drug therapy.

Drugs to avoid: Several AAD as well as noncardiac drugs may have a pro-arrhythmic effect in this group of disease. Arrhythmias are due to the effects of drugs on ion channels (with worse harm for potassium channel blockers in LQTS and sodium channel blockers in Brugada), that is, a target effect in AAD and a collateral effect of several other compounds. These drugs should be avoided or discontinued as a principal part of acute arrhythmia management in channelopa-thies; two panels of experts have created a web-based platform reporting and periodically updating all drugs that should be avoided in LQTS and Brugada syndrome: www.crediblemeds.org and www.brugadadrugs.org, respectively [18, 19, 26, 45].

These websites should be promptly consulted while managing these patients, mostly in emergency setting. In SQTS, at present, only one drug is known to have pro-arrhythmic effect and should be avoided (rufinamide, an antiepileptic drug), but other molecules may shorten QT in experimental isolated hearts and the list could grow in the future. *Electrolyte* abnormalities should be corrected (see Chap. 8) and sometimes overcorrected: *Potassium* repletion to 4.5–5 mmol/L may be considered for patients who present with torsades de pointes [31]; in CPVT patients calcium should not be administered.

Management with intravenous *magnesium sulfate* is reasonable for patients who present with *LQTS* and episodes of *torsades de pointes*. *Beta-blockers* can be com-bined with pacing for patients who present with TdP and sinus bradycardia [31]. In LQT3 intravenous *lidocaine or oral mexiletine* may be considered.

Acute drug therapy of *polymorphic ventricular arrhythmia in Brugada* syn-drome is based on isoproterenol infusion which increases the L-type calcium cur-rents (1–2 µg bolus i.v. followed by continuous infusion of 0.15–2.0 µg/min) and/or quinidine (300–1500 mg/day) [18, 21, 26]; quinidine is also useful for atrial fibril-lation in Brugada patients and should be considered in chronic prevention of recur-rences of both atrial and ventricular arrhythmias [4, 18, 21, 45]. Electrical storm in patients with early repolarization syndrome has to be managed by *isoproterenol infusion* (initiated at 1 µg/min targeting a 20 % increase in heart rate or an absolute heart rate >90 bpm, titrated to hemodynamic response, and suppression of recurrent ventricular arrhythmia); *quinidine* can be helpful for acute and long-term treatment [4, 32].

In CPVT patients therapy of acute ventricular arrhythmias is mainly based in adrenergic suppression; *verapamil* i.v. could be of use for short-term therapy [4, 16, 33].

8.3 What Cardiologists Should Know

Cardiologist should be promptly involved in the management of "channelopathy patients" in the setting of acute arrhythmias in order to:

1. Rule out structural heart disease and secondary causes that mimic channelopathies.
2. Define diagnosis.
3. Provide risk stratification in order to plan long-term management.

Diagnosis in channelopathies is essentially 12-lead ECG based, and more than 1 recording is usually indicated; triggering conditions could give a clue. *LQTS* diagnosis is based on QT measurement [34] corrected with Bazett formula: a QTc value ≥480 ms in repeated 12-lead ECG is diagnostic [45]; LQTS is diagnosed also in the presence of a risk score ≥3 [4, 35, 36, 45] or in the presence of an unequivocally pathogenic mutation in one of the LQTS genes. LQTS can be diagnosed in patients with QTc > or = 460 ms and unexplained syncope in the absence of secondary causes [4, 45].

Most arrhythmic events occur during physical or emotional stress in LQT1, at rest or in association with sudden noise in LQT2, and at rest or during sleep in LQT3 [37].

The use of provocative tests have been proposed to unmask LQTS in patients with normal QTc at resting ECG, like measurement during change from supine to standing position, in the recovery phase of exercise testing; clinical use of epinephrine for unmasking LQTS, however, is not unequivocally accepted [4].

SQTS is diagnosed in the presence of QTc ≤340 ms and diagnosis should be considered if QTc ≤360 ms in the presence of a pathogenic mutation or family history of SQTS/SCD at age <40 years or a VT or VF episode in the absence of heart disease [4, 45]. In one of the largest published SQTS series, it is reported that more than 60 % of the subjects had symptoms at presentation: cardiac arrest, the first clinical manifestation in one third of the patients, can occur in children during first year of life and in males between the second and fourth decade; syncope is the second most frequent clinical manifestation (15 % of cases). Events may occur both at rest and during effort, so it is not possible to identify a uniform trigger.

Brugada syndrome is diagnosed when a type 1 ST segment elevation is observed in at least one right precordial lead placed in a standard or superior position (up to the 2nd intercostal space) spontaneously or after intravenous administration of a sodium channel-blocking agent, as aymaline or flecainide [4, 9–11, 45]. Arrhythmic events typically occur during sleep or vagal stimulation. Risk stratification is based on the presence of spontaneous type 1 pattern and symptoms; there is no consensus on the value of electrophysiologic study in predicting long-term arrhythmic events [4].

CPVT is diagnosed in the presence of unexplained exercise or catecholamine-induced bidirectional or polymorphic ventricular tachycardia in individual without structural heart disease and with normal resting ECG [45]. In individuals >40 years of age, it can be diagnosed, but in this population, coronary artery disease should be excluded. CPVT is also diagnosed in patients with a pathogenic mutation [4, 45]. Arrhythmic events are typically induced by exercise and emotional stress and since basal ECG is usually normal and exercise stress test and loop recorders are pivotal investigations for diagnosis [4].

8.4   A Possible Algorithm/Pathway for Diagnosis and Treatment (Fig. 8.1; Table 8.1)

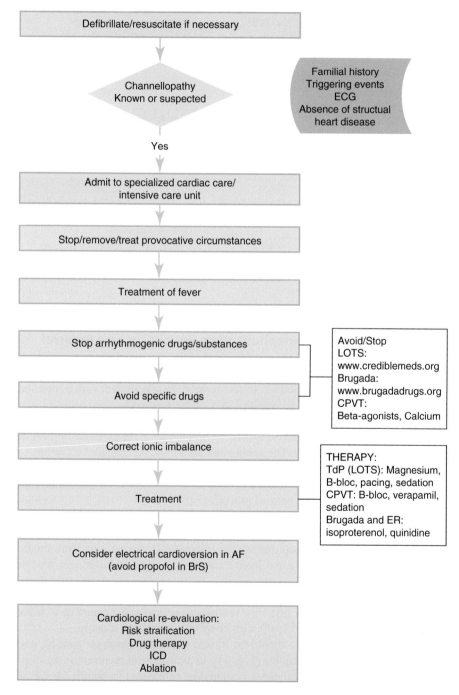

Fig. 8.1 A possible algorithm/pathway for diagnosis and treatment of arrhythmias in patients with channelopathies

Table 8.1 Conditions that can cause PVT/VF and potential therapies

Clues	Test to consider	Diagnoses	Therapies
Long QT/T wave alternans TdP History of seizures Specific triggers (loud noise)	ECG/monitor Epinephrine challenge Exercise stress test Genetic testing	Congenital LQTS	Beta-blockers Avoid QT-prolonging drugs In LQT3: mexiletine/flecainide PM/ICD Stellatectomy
Incomplete RBBB with STE in leads V1–V2 Fever	ECG Drug challenge Genetic testing	BrS	Isoproterenol/quinidine Antipyretic Ablation ICD
J-point elevation	ECG	Early repolarization	ICD
Short QT interval	ECG	SQTS	ICD Quinidine or sotalol
Bidirectional VT exercise induced	Exercise stress test Genetic testing	CPVT Andersen-Tawil syndrome	Beta-blockers/flecainide/verapamil ICD

Adapted from [15]: with permission

8.5 Indications for Hospitalization, Follow-Up, and Referral

Following the arrhythmic index event, channelopathy patient should be reevaluated for risk stratification and prevention of recurrences. Expert centers with a focus on inherited arrhythmias should be involved in complex cases [4].

Atrial arrhythmias in low-risk patients could be managed in out-of-hospital setting with referral to arrhythmia experts to set up indication for pharmacological or non-pharmacological strategy. Thromboembolism should be managed according to AF guidelines using CHA_2DS_2VASC score [20]. First line therapy consists in avoiding potentially pro-arrhythmic drugs and conditions: a complete list should be supplied to the patient and to the general practitioner.

CPVT and LQT patients should be advised to limit/avoid competitive sport, strenuous exercise, and exposure to stressful environments (which in LQT2 should include exposure to loud/abrupt noises, i.e., alarm bell); Brugada patients should avoid excessive alcohol intake and large meals and should be advised to a prompt treatment of fever [45].

Syncope and life-threatening arrhythmias require hospitalization.

Aborted sudden death and sustained ventricular arrhythmias require an ICD for secondary prevention [4, 15, 31, 45] with or without adjunctive therapy.

CPVT and LQTS patients should be treated with *beta-blockers: nadolol and propranolol* are the drugs of choice [1, 4, 33]; in patients with recurrent symptoms/arrhythmias already on beta-blockers, it should be considered *flecainide for CPVT*

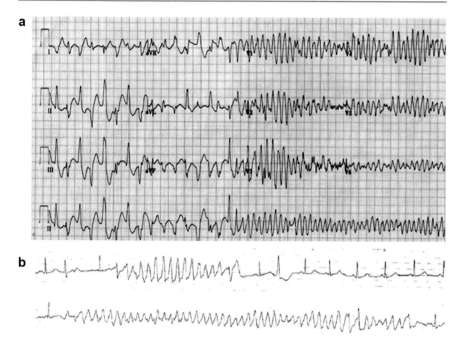

Fig. 8.2 Panel (**a**):12-lead ECG from a 9-year-old boy with ryanodine-positive CPVT shows a transition from triggered bidirectional ventricular tachycardia followed by brief polymorphic ventricular tachycardia to reentrant ventricular fibrillation. With permission from Elsevier Roses-Noguer F. et al. [43]: Copyright © 2014 Heart Rhythm Society. Panel (**b**): torsades de point. With permission from Van der Heide et al. [44]

patients [33] and *flecainide or ranolazine or mexiletine in LQT3* patients [4]; ICD and left cardiac denervation should be considered in patients refractory to pharmacological therapy [4, 33]. Repeated exercise stress test is used in CPVT patients to evaluate drug efficacy.

Brugada and SQTS patients symptomatic for syncope should be treated with *ICD*; quinidine therapy could be used as adjunctive therapy or in cases in which ICD is refused or contraindicated or in recurrent appropriate ICD intervention [22, 26].

Hydroquinidine has proven to play a role in AF recurrence prevention in Brugada patients [4, 21].

Refractory electrical storm could be evaluated for catheter ablation of triggers [15, 39–41, 45].

All clinically diagnosed patients with LQTS and CPVT should undergo *genetic evaluation* if not previously performed, and it can be useful in Brugada (type1) patients and SQTS [42]. Routine genetic testing is not indicated for the survivor of an unexplained out-of-hospital cardiac arrest in the absence of a clinical index of suspicion for a specific cardiomyopathy or channelopathy [42] (Figs. 8.2 and 8.3)

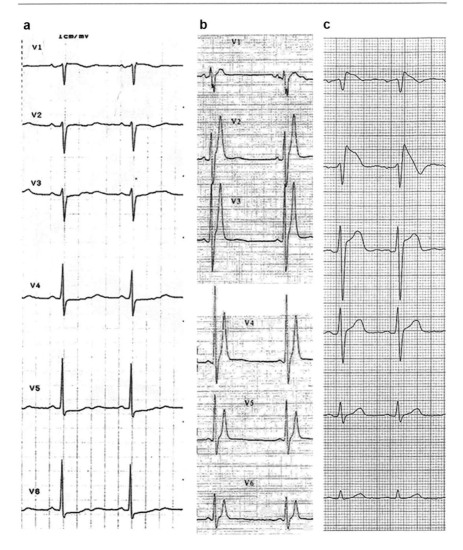

Fig. 8.3 Precordial leads ECG in patients with panel (**a**), long QT syndrome, heart rate 58 beats per minute, QTc 600 ms; panel (**b**), short QT syndrome, heart rate 52 beats per minute (bpm), QT 280 ms*; panel (**c**), Brugada syndrome, coved ST elevation in V1–V2. *With permission from Gaita F. et al. [7]

References

1. Cerrone M, Priori SG. Genetics of sudden death: focus on inherited channelopathies. Eur Heart J. 2011;32:2109–18.
2. Patel C, Burke JF, Patel H, et al. Is there a significant transmural gradient in repolarization time in the intact heart? Cellular basis of the T wave: a century of controversy. Circ Arrhythm Electrophysiol. 2009;2(1):80–8.

3. Hocini M, Pison L, Proclemer A, et al. Diagnosis and management of patients with inherited arrhythmias in Europe: results of the European Heart Rhythm Association Survey. Europace. 2014;16:600–3.
4. Priori SG, Wilde AA, Horie M, et al. HRS/EHRA/APHRS expert consensus statement on the diagnosis and management of patients with inherited primary arrhythmia syndromes. Heart Rhythm. 2013;10(12):1932–63.
5. Moss AJ. Long QT syndrome. JAMA. 2003;289:2041–4.
6. Campuzano O, Allegue C, Fernandez A, et al. Determining the pathogenicity of genetic variants associated with cardiac channelopathies. Sci Rep. 2015;7953:1–6.
7. Gaita F, Giustetto C, Bianchi F, et al. Short QT syndrome: a familial cause of sudden death. Circulation. 2003;108(8):965–70.
8. Giustetto C, Schimpf R, Mazzanti A, et al. Long-term follow-up of patients with short QT syndrome. J Am Coll Cardiol. 2011;58(6):587–95.
9. Antzelevitch C, Brugada P, Borggrefe M, et al. Brugada syndrome: report of the Second Consensus Conference: Endorsed by the Heart Rhythm Society and the European Heart Rhythm Association. Circulation. 2005;111:659–70.
10. Bayés de Luna A, Brugada J, Baranchuk A, et al. Current electrocardiographic criteria for diagnosis of brugada pattern: a consensus report. J Electrocardiol. 2012;45(5):433.
11. Berne P, Brugada J. Brugada syndrome. Circ J. 2012;76:1563–71.
12. Priori SG, Napolitano C, Memmi M, et al. Clinical and molecular characterization of patients with catecholaminergic polymorphic ventricular tachycardia. Circulation. 2002;106:69.
13. Haissaguerre M, Sacher F, Nogami A, et al. Characteristics of recurrent ventricular fibrillation associated with inferolateral early repolarization role of drug therapy. J Am Coll Cardiol. 2009;53(7):612–9.
14. Mahida S, Derval N, Sacher F, et al. Role of electrophysiological studies in predicting risk of ventricular arrhythmia in early repolarization syndrome. J Am Coll Cardiol. 2015;65(2):151.159.
15. Pedersen CT, Kay GN, Kalman J, et al. EHRA/HRS/APHRS expert consensus on ventricular arrhythmias. Heart Rhythm. 2014;11(10):e166–96.
16. Leenhardt A, Lucet V, Denjoy I, et al. Catecholaminergic polymorphic ventricular tachycardia in children : a 7-year follow-up of 21 patients. Circulation. 1995;91(5):1512–9.
17. Dessertenne F. Ventricular tachycardia with two variable opposing foci. Arch Mal Coeur Vaiss. 1966;59:263–72.
18. Postema PG, Neville J, de Jong JS, et al. Safe drug use in long QT syndrome and brugada syndrome: comparison of website statistics. Europace. 2013;15:1042–9.
19. Drew BJ, Ackerman MJ, Funk M, et al. Prevention of Torsade de Pointes in Hospital Settings. J Am Coll Cardiol. 2010;55:934–47.
20. January CT, Wann LS, Alpert JS, et al. AHA/ACC/HRS guideline for the management of patients with atrial fibrillation. Circulation. 2014;130(23):2071–104.
21. Giustetto C, Cerrato N, Gribaudo E, et al. Atrial fibrillation in a large population with Brugada electrocardiographic pattern: prevalence, management, and correlation with prognosis. Heart Rhythm. 2014;11:259–65.
22. Chen YH, Xu SJ, Bedahlou S, et al. KCNQ1 gain-of-function mutation in familial atrial fibrillation. Science. 2003;299:251–4.
23. Johnson JN, et al. Prevalence of early-onset atrial fibrillation in congenital long QT syndrome. Heart Rhythm. 2008;5(5):704–9.
24. Zellerhoff S, Pistulli R, Mönnig G, et al. Atrial arrhythmias in long-QT syndrome under daily life conditions: a nested case control study. J Cardiovasc Electrophysiol. 2009;20(4):401–7.
25. Schimpf R, Wolpert C, Bianchi F, et al. "Congenital" short QT syndrome and implantable cardioverter defibrillator treatment: inherent risk for inappropriate shock delivery. J Cardiovasc Electrophysiol. 2003;14:1–5.
26. Postema PG, Wolpert C, Amin AS, et al. Drugs and Brugada syndrome patients: review of the literature, recommendations, and an up-to-date website (www.brugadadrugs.org). Heart Rhythm. 2009;6:1335–41.

27. Amin AS, Meregalli PG, Bardai A, et al. Fever increases the risk for cardiac arrest in the Brugada syndrome. Ann Intern Med. 2008;149:216–8.
28. Burashnikov A, Wataru Shimizu W, Antzelevitch C. Fever accentuates transmural dispersion of repolarization and facilitates the development of early afterdepolarizations and torsade de pointes under long QT conditions. Circ Arrhythm Electrophysiol. 2008;1(3):202–8.
29. Amin AS, Herfst LJ, Delisle BP, et al. Fever-induced QTc prolongation and ventricular arrhythmias in type 2 congenital long QT. J Clin Invest. 2008;118(7):2552–61.
30. Shen MJ, Zipes DP. Role of the autonomic nervous system in modulating cardiac arrhythmias. Circ Res. 2014;114:1004–21.
31. Zipes DP, Camm AJ, Borggrefe M, et al. ACC/AHA/ESC 2006 guidelines for management of patients with ventricular arrhythmias and the prevention of sudden cardiac death. J Am Coll Cardiol. 2006;48:e247–346.
32. Nam GB, Kim YH, Antzelevich C. Augmentation of J waves and electrical storms in patients with early repolarization. N Engl J Med. 2008;358(19):2078–9.
33. van der Werf C, Zwinderman AH, Wilde AAM. Therapeutic approach for patients with catecholaminergic polymorphic ventricular tachycardia: state of the art and future developments. Europace. 2012;14:175–83.
34. Postema PG, De Jong JSSG, Van der Bilt IAC, Wilde AAM. Accurate electrocardiographic assessment of the QT interval: Teach the tangent. Heart Rhythm. 2008;5(7):1015–8.
35. Schwartz PJ, Crotti L. QTc behavior during exercise and genetic testing for the long QT syndrome. Circulation. 2011;124(20):2181–4.
36. Schwartz PJ, Moss AJ, Vincent GM. Diagnostic criteria for the long QT syndrome. An update. Circulation. 1993;88(2):782–4.
37. Schwartz PJ, Priori SG, Spazzolini C, et al. Genotype-phenotype correlation in the long-QT syndrome: gene-specific triggers for life-threatening arrhythmias. Circulation. 2011;103(1):89–95.
38. Veltmann C, Borggrefe M. Arrhythmias: a "Schwartz score" for short QT syndrome. Nat Rev Cardiol. 2011;8(5):251–2.
39. Haissaguerre M, Extramiana F, Hocini M, Cauchemez B, Jaïs P, Cabrera JA, et al. Mapping and ablation of ventricular fibrillation associated with long-QT and brugada syndromes. Circulation. 2003;108(8):925–8.
40. Nademanee K, Veerakul G, Chandanamattha P, Chaothawee L, Ariyachaipanich A, Jirasirirojanakorn K, et al. Prevention of ventricular fibrillation episodes in Brugada syndrome by catheter ablation over the anterior right ventricular outflow tract epicardium. Circulation. 2011;123:1270–9.
41. Willems S, Hoffmann BA, Schaeffer B, Sultan A, Schreiber D, Lüker J, Steven D. Mapping and ablation of ventricular fibrillation—how and for whom? J Interv Card Electrophysiol. 2014;40:229–35.
42. Ackerman MJ, Priori SG, Willems S, et al. HRS/EHRA expert consensus statement on the state of genetic testing for the channelopathies and cardiomyopathies. Europace. 2011;13:1077–109.
43. Roses-Noguer F, Jarman JWE, Clague JR, Till J. Outcomes of defibrillator therapy in catecholaminergic polymorphic ventricular tachycardia. Heart Rhythm. 2014;11(1):58–66.
44. Van der Heide K, de Haes A, Wietasch GJK, Wiesfeld ACP, Hendriks HGD. Torsades de pointes during laparoscopic adrenalectomy of a pheochromocytoma: a case report. J Med Case Rep. 2011;5:368.
45. Priori SG, Blomstrom-Lunqvist C, Mazzanti A, et al. 2015 ESCA Guidelines for the management of patients with ventricular arrhythmias and the prevention of sudden cardiac death. Eur Heart J 2015 Aug 29. PMID 26320108

Acute Management of Patients with Arrhythmias and Non-cardiac Diseases: Metabolite Disorders and Ion Disturbances

Stefano Bardari, Biancamaria D'Agata, and Gianfranco Sinagra

9.1 Focusing on the Issue

Acute metabolic disorders are relatively common amongst medical and surgical patients, especially if critically ill. Whilst increasing the complexity of management plans, these circumstances also increase the risk of cardiac complications, such as arrhythmias, and furthermore are associated with increased mortality. Arrhythmic risk is promoted by electrolyte, acid-base and fluid balance disturbance, increased sympathetic drive and cardiac ischaemia. Particularly, electrolyte abnormalities may generate or facilitate clinical arrhythmias, even in the setting of normal cardiac tissue, by modulating ion conduction across (specific) cardiac cell membrane channels [1], and management of the underlying pathology may be all that is required to allow rapid normalisation of the metabolic profile. Moreover, complex pharmacological regimes may exacerbate the situation [2].

9.1.1 Metabolite Disorders

Endocrine disorders can induce ventricular tachycardia (VT) and sudden cardiac death (SCD) by excess or insufficient hormonal activity on myocardial receptors (e.g. pheochromocytoma, hypothyroidism). The endocrinopathy can also cause myocardial changes (e.g. acromegaly) or electrolyte disturbances produced by

S. Bardari (✉)
Cardiology Unit, Gorizia Hospital, AAS 2 Bassa Friulana - Isontina, Gorizia, Italy
e-mail: stefanobardari@hotmail.it

B. D'Agata
Institute for Maternal and Child Health-IRCCS, Burlo Garofalo, University of Trieste, Trieste, Italy

G. Sinagra
Cardiovascular Department, Ospedali Riuniti and University of Trieste, Trieste, Italy

© Springer International Publishing Switzerland 2016
M. Zecchin, G. Sinagra (eds.), *The Arrhythmic Patient in the Emergency Department: A Practical Guide for Cardiologists and Emergency Physicians*,
DOI 10.1007/978-3-319-24328-3_9

129

hormone excess (e.g. hyperkalaemia in Addison disease and hypokalaemia in Conn syndrome), and certain endocrine disorders can accelerate the progression of conditions such as underlying structural heart disease secondary to dyslipidaemia or hypertension, increasing the risk of serious arrhythmias [3].

In addition to electrolyte shifts and ischemia, other systemic influences found in the critically ill patient, such as acid-base abnormalities, hypoxia and enhanced catecholamine levels, can also predispose to ventricular arrhythmias [4]. The mechanism of these arrhythmias is due to automaticity or triggered activity through stimulation of the β-adrenergic receptor, sympathetic activation or exogenous catecholamines. Re-entry may also be facilitated, particularly in the presence of ischemia [5]. The management of ventricular arrhythmias secondary to endocrine disorders should address the electrolyte (potassium, magnesium and calcium) imbalance and the treatment of the underlying endocrinopathy.

9.1.1.1 Thyroid Disorders

Thyrotoxicosis commonly causes atrial arrhythmias; cases of VT/SCD are extremely uncommon but may occur with concomitant electrolyte disturbances. VT/SCD is more common in hypothyroidism, the basic underlying mechanism being possibly related to prolongation of the QT interval [6, 7]. Thyroxin replacement therapy usually corrects this abnormality and prevents any further arrhythmias, but antiarrhythmic drugs, such as procainamide, have been used successfully in an emergency.

9.1.1.2 Phaeochromocytoma

Phaeochromocytoma may present with VT/SCD, but there are no data to quantify its incidence, best mode of management or response to treatment. Conventional antagonism of catecholamine excess with α-receptor blockers followed by β-blockade helps control hypertension and reverses or prevents any further structural deterioration [8], but there is only anecdotal evidence that it prevents recurrence of ventricular arrhythmia [9]. Early definite surgical treatment of the phaeochromocytoma should be a priority, especially in cases with documented life-threatening arrhythmias. In some patients with VT associated with phaeochromocytoma, a long QT interval has been identified [10, 11].

9.1.1.3 Acromegaly

SCD is an established manifestation of acromegaly, and life-threatening arrhythmias are likely to be an important cause [12]. Up to one half of all acromegalic patients have complex ventricular arrhythmias on 24-h Holter recordings, and of these, approximately two thirds are repetitive [13]. Appropriate surgical management of the pituitary tumour is paramount for improved long-term outcome, as cardiac changes are reversible, especially in the young [14, 15]. Somatostatin analogues such as octreotide and lanreotide have both been shown to improve the ventricular arrhythmia profile [16–18].

9.1.1.4 Primary Aldosteronism, Addison Disease, Hyperparathyroidism and Hypoparathyroidism

Severe electrolyte disturbances form the basis of arrhythmogenesis and VT/SCD associated with the previously mentioned endocrinopathies. Electrocardiographic (ECG) changes including prolongation of QRS and QTc intervals can accompany the electrolyte disturbance. Electrolyte imbalance requires immediate attention before definitive treatment of the underlying cause [19–21].

9.1.1.5 Diabetic Ketoacidosis (DKA)

As its name suggests, DKA is defined by the presence of metabolic acidosis, along with hyperglycaemia, as a result of insulin deficiency. These factors are generally accompanied by severe dehydration, catecholamine release and disordered potassium homeostasis; deviation of magnesium, sodium and other electrolytes can also occur. The syndrome is most often precipitated by sepsis or poor medication compliance with direct cardiac consequences, such as arrhythmias [22]. With appropriate insulin and fluid therapy, the acidosis is reversed and concomitantly potassium is forced into cells, often resulting in rebound hypokalaemia. Without frequent biochemical monitoring, such dynamic metabolic changes may deviate from normality without being acted upon, so increasing the likelihood of cardiac compromise.

During the acute phase of treatment, the rapid transition of potassium gradients changes the type of arrhythmia susceptibility. Initially, hyperkalaemia slows conduction and normal automaticity favouring bradycardias, re-entrant VT and ventricular fibrillation (VF). Later, hypokalaemia favours re-entrant arrhythmias, polymorphic VT and atrial fibrillation (AF) due to triggered activity. However, the broader spectrum of dynamic metabolic changes present in DKA will also impact upon the risk of arrhythmia, potentially through complex interactions between all of the mechanisms outlined earlier. This has led to recommendations of continuous electrocardiographic monitoring during the acute phase of treatment, although the evidence of benefit for this as a routine approach is lacking [23].

9.1.2 Ion Disturbances

Electrolyte abnormalities are commonly associated with cardiovascular emergencies. These abnormalities are amongst the most common causes of cardiac arrhythmias, and they can (cause or) complicate resuscitation attempts and post-resuscitation care. If extreme, even isolated electrolyte deficiency or excess can cause life-threatening cardiac involvement in patients with structurally normal hearts. Clinical syndromes that create hypo- and hyper-concentrations of potassium, calcium and magnesium are associated with the most common and clinically important disturbances of cardiac rhythm related to electrolyte abnormality. Despite the frequency of sodium abnormalities, particularly hyponatraemia, its electrophysiological effects are rarely clinically significant. It is important to identify clinical situations in which electrolyte problems may be expected. In some cases therapy for life-threatening electrolyte disorders should be initiated even before laboratory results become available. Of all the electrolyte abnormalities, hyperkalaemia is the most rapidly fatal. A high degree of clinical suspicion and aggressive treatment of underlying electrolyte abnormalities can prevent these abnormalities from progressing to cardiac arrest [24]. Electrocardiographic findings associated with these disturbances can provide clues to the diagnosis as well as guide therapeutic interventions. Although discussed individually, it is important to remember that there is a dynamic physiologic interrelationship to electrolyte homeostasis and that aberration in one 'compartment' may have impact on another [25].

9.1.2.1 Potassium

Potassium (K$^+$) is the most abundant intracellular cation with only 2 % of the total body potassium in the extracellular space, and hypokalaemia is the most common electrolyte abnormality in clinical practice. Potassium plays an important role in maintaining the electrical potential across the cellular membrane as well as in depolarisation and repolarisation of the myocytes. The electrophysiological effects of potassium depend not only on its extracellular concentration but also on the direction (hypokalaemia *vs* hyperkalaemia) and rate of change. Although the mechanism of potassium regulation between compartments is complex, there are two main transport processes. An active transport process involves the Na$^+$/K$^+$ ATPase pump, insulin, beta-adrenergic agents and mineral corticosteroids and a passive transport that results from alterations in the pH and extracellular cellular fluid osmolality. Homeostatic serum potassium concentration is maintained by terminal nephron segments of the kidney. Factors that lead to alterations in serum potassium regulation include renal failure and medications such as non-steroidal anti-inflammatory agents, angiotensin-converting enzyme inhibitors, diuretics and digitalis [26, 27]. Alterations in serum potassium levels can have dramatic effects on cardiac cell conduction and may lead to EKG changes, and the electrocardiogram is a useful screening tool for gauging the severity of the serum potassium abnormality and the urgency of therapeutic intervention [28, 29].

Hyperkalaemia

Hyperkalaemia is a common disorder, although less common than hypokalaemia, occurring both in the outpatient setting and in up to 8 % of patients who have been admitted to hospital, mainly in the setting of compromised renal function [30–33]. Hyperkalaemia is defined as an excess concentration of potassium ions in the extracellular fluid compartment above the normal range of 3.5–5.0 mEq/L. Moderate (6–7 mEq/L) and severe (>7 mEq/L) hyperkalaemia is life-threatening and requires immediate therapy. Although mild hyperkalaemia is often asymptomatic and easily treated, acute and severe hyperkalaemia, if left untreated, can result in fatal cardiac arrhythmias [34–36].

The most common clinical presentation of severe hyperkalaemia involves patients with end-stage renal failure. Identification of potential causes of hyperkalaemia will contribute to rapid identification and treatment of patients who may be experiencing hyperkalaemic cardiac arrhythmias [37–39]. Potassium-sparing diuretics such as spironolactone, triamterene and amiloride are well-recognised causes of hyperkalaemia. Use of angiotensin-converting enzyme (ACE) inhibitors can also lead to elevation of serum potassium, particularly when combined with oral potassium supplements. Moreover, non-steroidal anti-inflammatory medicines can cause hyperkalaemia through direct effects on the kidney.

Physical symptoms of hyperkalaemia include weakness, ascending paralysis and respiratory failure.

Electrocardiographic manifestations of hyperkalaemia. The EKG manifestation of hyperkalaemia depends on serum K$^+$ level. Studies validate a good correlation with hyperkalaemia and EKG changes, but 50 % of patients with potassium levels greater than 6.5 mEq/L will not manifest any ECG changes.

The increased extracellular concentration of K$^+$ causes an influx of K$^+$ into the cells. There is an alteration of the transmembrane potential gradient, a decrease in magnitude of the resting potential and a decrease in velocity of phase 0 of the action potential. The K^+ influx causes a shortening of the action potential and results in delayed conduction between the myocytes and ECG change, such as the *T wave tenting*, classically described as symmetrically narrow or peaked, though the deflection is often wide and of large amplitude [40]. In addition, inverted T waves associated with left ventricular hypertrophy can *pseudonormalise* (i.e., flip upright) [41]. These T wave changes occur as a result of the acceleration of the terminal phase of repolarisation, are most prominently seen in the precordial leads and are often seen when potassium levels exceed *5.5 mEq/L*. With higher levels of serum potassium, cardiac conduction between myocytes is suppressed. Reduction in atrial and ventricular transmembrane potential causes an inactivation of the sodium channel, decreasing the cellular action potential. Atrial tissue is more sensitive to these changes earlier, and, as a result, P wave flattening and PR interval prolongation may be seen before QRS interval prolongation. These changes generally occur when potassium levels exceed *6.5 mEq/L* [42]. As the serum level continues to rise to levels above *twice the normal value*, there is suppression of sinoatrial and atrioventricular conduction, resulting in sinoatrial and atrioventricular blocks, often with escape beats. Other blocks including intraventricular conduction delay, bundle branch block and fascicular blocks have been reported. The bundle branch blocks associated with hyperkalaemia are atypical in the sense that they involve the initial and terminal forces of the QRS complex. Shifts in the QRS axis indicate disproportionate conduction delays in the left bundle fascicles [43]. As hyperkalaemia progresses, depolarisation merges with repolarisation, expressed in the ECG with *QT shortening* and *apparent ST segment elevation* simulating acute injury [44]. Atypical bundle branch blocks (LBBB and RBBB), intraventricular conduction delays, VT, ventricular fibrillation and idioventricular rhythm are more commonly seen in cases of severe hyperkalaemia.

Hypokalaemia

Hypokalaemia, defined as a serum potassium level *<3.5 mEq/L*, is the most common electrolyte abnormality encountered in clinical practice. It is observed in over 20 % of hospitalised patients [45], because of the high prevalence of patients on medications that can result in hypokalaemia, as 10–40 % of patients on thiazide diuretics have low potassium levels [46]; moreover, almost 50 % of patients resuscitated from out-of-hospital VF [47].

The most common causes of low serum potassium are gastrointestinal loss (diarrhoea, laxatives), renal loss (hyperaldosteronism), severe hyperglycaemia, potassium depleting, diuretics, carbenicillin, sodium penicillin, amphotericin B, intracellular shift (alkalosis or a rise in pH) and malnutrition.

The major consequences of severe hypokalaemia result from its effects on nerves and muscles (including the heart). The myocardium is extremely sensitive to the effects of hypokalaemia, particularly if the patient is taking a digitalis derivative. Symptoms of mild hypokalaemia are weakness, fatigue, paralysis, respiratory difficulty, constipation, paralytic ileus and leg cramps; more severe hypokalaemia will alter cardiac tissue excitability and conduction.

Electrocardiographic manifestations of hypokalaemia. In cases of severe hypokalaemia, EKG changes can be a very useful, quick, inexpensive and widely available diagnostic tool. The ECG manifestations of hypokalaemia [48] are due to its effects on repolarisation and conduction. As serum potassium levels decline, transmembrane potassium gradient decreases. The effect on cell membrane is elevation in resting membrane potential and prolongation of the action potential, particularly phase 3 repolarisation and refractory periods.

The *earliest ECG change* associated with hypokalaemia is a *decrease in the T wave amplitude*.

As potassium *levels further decline, ST segment depression and T wave inversions* can be seen and the *U wave becomes more prominent*. The *PR interval can be prolonged,* and there can be an *increase in the amplitude of the P wave*.

With *even lower serum potassium levels*, the classic ECG change associated with hypokalaemia is the development of *U waves*. The U wave is described as a positive deflection after the T wave that is often best seen in the mid-precordial leads, such as V2 and V3. These changes have been reported in almost 80 % of patients with potassium levels <2.7 mEq/L [49].

With *extreme hypokalaemia, giant U waves* may often mask the smaller preceding T waves or following P waves [50]. The characteristic reversal in the relative amplitude of the T and U waves is the most distinctive change in waveform morphology in hypokalaemia. The U wave in hypokalaemia is caused by prolongation of the recovery phase of the cardiac potential, the relative refractory period predisposing to re-entrant tachyarrhythmias.

Magnesium

Although magnesium is the fourth most common mineral and the second most abundant intracellular cation (after potassium) in the human body, the significance of magnesium disorders is controversial partly because of the frequent association of other electrolyte abnormalities. Magnesium is an important cofactor in several enzymatic reactions contributing to normal cardiovascular physiology.

The average adult contains about 24 g of magnesium, with only 1 % found in the extracellular space [51]. One third of extracellular magnesium is bound to serum albumin. Therefore, serum magnesium levels are not reliable predictors of total body magnesium stores. It plays an important role in stabilising excitable membranes and may influence the incidence of cardiac arrhythmias through a direct effect, by modulating the effects of potassium, or through its action as a calcium channel blocker. Magnesium deficiency is thought to interfere with the normal functioning of membrane ATPase and thus the pumping of sodium out of the cell and potassium into the cell [52].

Hypermagnesaemia. Hypermagnesaemia is defined as a serum magnesium concentration *>2.2 mEq/L* (normal: 1.3–2.2 mEq/L). Magnesium balance is influenced by many of the same regulatory systems that control calcium balance and by diseases and factors that control serum potassium. As a result, magnesium balance is closely tied to both calcium and potassium balance. The most common cause of hypermagnesaemia is renal failure. Hypermagnesaemia may also be iatrogenic (caused by overuse of magnesium) or caused by continued use of laxatives or antacids containing magnesium (an important cause in the elderly). Severe symptoms include neurological symptoms, areflexia, muscular weakness, paralysis, ataxia, drowsiness, confusion, respiratory failure and, rarely, cardiac arrest. Gastrointestinal symptoms include nausea and vomiting. Moderate hypermagnesaemia can produce vasodilation, and severe hypermagnesaemia can produce hypotension. Extremely high serum magnesium levels may produce a depressed level of consciousness, bradycardia, hypoventilation and cardiorespiratory arrest [53].

Electrocardiographic manifestations of hypermagnesaemia. ECG changes of hypermagnesaemia include the following:

- Increased QRS duration
- Increased PR and QT intervals
- Variable decrease in P wave voltage
- Variable degree of T wave peaking
- Complete AV block and asystole

Hypomagnesaemia. Hypomagnesaemia, defined as a serum magnesium concentration <1.3 mEq/L, is far more common than hypermagnesaemia. It is caused by decreased intake, increased losses or altered intracellular-extracellular distribution. Hypomagnesaemia usually results from decreased absorption or increased loss, either from the kidneys or intestines (diarrhoea). Alterations in parathyroid hormone and certain medications (e.g. pentamidine, diuretics, alcohol) can also induce hypomagnesaemia. Lactating women are at higher risk of developing hypomagnesaemia.

Measurement of serum levels do not correlate well with clinical manifestations. Hypomagnesaemia is associated with far-reaching adversity across the physiologic spectrum, including central nervous system effects (seizures, mental status changes), cardiovascular effects (dysrhythmias, vasospasm), endocrine effects (hypokalaemia, hypocalcaemia) and muscle effect (bronchospasm, muscle weakness) [54].

Electrocardiographic manifestations of hypomagnesaemia. A number of ECG abnormalities occur with low magnesium levels, including the following:

- ST segment depression
- Prolonged QT and PR intervals
- T wave inversion
- Flattening or inversion of precordial P waves
- Widening of QRS
- Torsades de pointes, treatment-resistant VF (and other arrhythmias) and worsening of digitalis toxicity [55]

Calcium

Calcium (Ca^{++}) is the most abundant mineral in the body. It is essential for bone strength and neuromuscular function and plays a major role in myocardial contraction. The human body has a nearly inexhaustible reservoir of Ca^{++} stored as hydroxyapatite in skeletal bone. Of the total 1–2 kg of adult total body Ca^{++}, only 1 g of calcium is present in plasma. Ca^{++} is important in a myriad of regulatory mechanisms, skeletal muscle contraction and control of enzymatic reactions and is a key ion in myocyte electrical activity and myocardial contraction [56]. Although total serum calcium Ca^{++} is directly related to serum albumin, the ionised Ca^{++} is inversely related to serum albumin. The lower the serum albumin, the higher the ionised calcium. Isolated abnormalities of extracellular Ca^{++} produce clinically significant electrophysiological effects only when they are extreme in either direction.

Hypercalcaemia. Hypercalcaemia is defined as a serum Ca^{++} concentration above the normal range of 8.5–10.5 mEq/L (or an elevation in ionised calcium above 4.2–4.8 mg/dL).

Hypercalcaemia is the cardinal feature of *hyperparathyroidism.* Primary hyperparathyroidism and malignancy account for >90 % of reported cases [57]. It is typically chronic, mild and well tolerated. Severe hypercalcaemia with serum levels *above 14 mg/dL* can be precipitated in these patients by dehydration from gastrointestinal losses, diuretic therapy or ingestion of large amounts of calcium salts.

Symptoms of hypercalcaemia usually develop when the total serum Ca^{++} concentration reaches or exceeds 12–15 mg/dL and can be relatively vague, including fatigue, lethargy, motor weakness, anorexia, nausea, constipation and abdominal pain. Effects on the kidney include diminished ability to concentrate urine; diuresis, leading to loss of sodium, potassium, magnesium and phosphate; and a vicious circle of calcium reabsorption that further worsens hypercalcaemia. At higher levels patients may exhibit hallucinations, disorientation, hypotonicity and coma. Cardiovascular symptoms of elevated Ca^{++} levels are variable. Myocardial contractility may initially increase until the Ca^{++} level reaches *15–20 mg/dL. Above* this level myocardial depression occurs. Automaticity is decreased, but arrhythmias occur because the refractory period is shortened, many patients develop hypokalaemia and digitalis toxicity is worsened [58].

Electrocardiographic manifestations of hypercalcaemia. The effect of hypercalcaemia on the electrocardiogram is the opposite of hypocalcaemia with the hallmark of abnormal shortening of the QTc interval. Cardiac conduction abnormalities may occur, with bradydysrhythmias being the most common [59]. ECG changes of hypercalcaemia include the following:

- Prolonged PR and QRS intervals
- Shortened QT interval (usually when Ca^{++} is >13 mg/dL)
- Increased QRS voltage with notching of QRS complex
- T wave flattening and widening
- AV block, progressing to complete heart block and to cardiac arrest when serum calcium is >15–20 mg/dL

Hypocalcaemia. Hypocalcaemia is defined as a serum calcium concentration below the normal range of 8.5–10.5 mg/dL (or an ionised calcium below the range of 4.2–4.8 mg/dL). Hypocalcaemia is classically seen with *functional parathyroid hormone deficiency,* either as absolute hormone deficiency (primary hypoparathyroidism), post-parathyroidectomy or related to a pseudo-hypoparathyroid syndrome. Other causes of hypocalcaemia include *vitamin D deficiency, congenital disorders of calcium metabolism, chronic renal failure, acute pancreatitis, rhabdomyolysis and sepsis.* Hypocalcaemia is commonly seen in critically ill patients, with a reported incidence of as high as 50 % [60]. Furthermore, hypocalcaemia is often associated with hypomagnesaemia. Symptoms usually occur when ionised levels fall *below 2.5 mg/dL.* Neuromuscular irritability is the cardinal feature, with carpal-pedal spasm being the classical physical sign that may progress to tetany, laryngo-spasm or hyperreflexia and positive Chvostek and Trousseau signs.

Hypocalcaemia prolongs phase 2 of the action potential. *Prolongation of the QTc interval* is associated with early after-repolarisations and triggered dysrhythmias. Torsades de pointes potentially can be triggered by hypocalcaemia but is much less common than with hypokalaemia or hypomagnesaemia.

Severe symptoms and life-threatening dysrhythmias mandate immediate treatment; in addition, associated electrolyte abnormalities, including hypomagnesaemia, phosphate abnormalities and acidemia, may need to be corrected.

Electrocardiographic manifestations of hypocalcaemia. Hypocalcaemia results in *prolonged ST segment and QT interval,* a potential cause of torsades de pointes, although much less commonly than with hypokalaemia or hypomagnesaemia [61]. Whereas electrocardiographic conduction abnormalities are common, serious hypocalcaemia-induced dysrhythmias such as heart block and ventricular dysrhythmias are infrequent.

9.1.2.2 Management of Arrhythmic Complications

Encountering a seriously ill patient with complex metabolic derangement and cardiac, or multi-organ, compromise can be daunting. Firstly, the basic principles of resuscitation provide a means of optimising basic cardiorespiratory physiology whilst giving time to consider the more complex metabolic needs of the patient. Depending on the underlying presentation or disorder, an appropriate initial assessment of electrolytes, acid-base and fluid balance status should be made. The results of this, in addition to the likelihood of rapid changes due to treatment or the natural history of the disorder, should be used to guide timing of repeat assessments. Furthermore, a strategy to normalise the patient's biochemical profile should be planned and regularly updated; addressing the underlying disorder may be all that is required in some cases. Where profound derangement is present, or when treatment of the underlying disease is failing to achieve the goal of physiological normalisation, it may be necessary to provide additional treatment targeted at specific metabolic parameters. This may involve electrolyte correction, rehydration and reduction of other factors, such as hypoxia, which worsens ischaemia. *Manipulation of acid-base status is generally not recommended* [62, 63]; in DKA, or other forms of acidosis, expert consensus suggests sodium bicarbonate therapy results in net harm, perhaps by worsening intracellular acidosis. Bicarbonate is still administered on occasions, but in the most profoundly acidotic patients and often as an act of desperation.

Unfortunately, the evidence base to guide such decisions is limited and so relies upon expert consensus. A 12-lead ECG with continuous recording of the rhythm strip provides invaluable information, but should not be allowed to interfere with emergent treatment where required. If the patient is 'compensating' haemodynamically for their rhythm disturbance, then time is available to classify the rhythm disturbance and manage according to accepted guidance [64]. It is crucial to remember that any 'antiarrhythmic' pharmacotherapy commenced may have unintended pro-arrhythmic consequences, particularly in the setting of metabolic abnormalities

[65]. The principle of never prescribing antiarrhythmic 'cocktails' is even more pertinent in this scenario.

Treatment of Hyperkalaemia

A variety of treatment options are considered for the acute management of hyperkalaemia, including insulin, β2-adrenergic agonists (inhaled, nebulised and intravenous), bicarbonate, resins, fludrocortisone, aminophylline and dialysis.

The treatment of hyperkalaemia is determined by its severity and the patient's clinical condition. First you need to stop the sources of exogenous potassium administration (e.g. consider supplements and maintenance IV fluids) and evaluate drugs that can increase serum potassium (e.g. potassium-sparing diuretics, ACE inhibitors, non-steroidal anti-inflammatory agents). The level of potassium at which treatment should be initiated has not been established by evidence. Several treatment options have been proposed, particularly for shifting potassium into the cells, with differing onset and duration of action [66].

For *mild* elevation *(5.5–6 mEq/L)*, remove potassium from the body with the following:

1. Diuretics—furosemide 1 mg/kg IV slowly
2. Resins—Kayexalate 15–30 g in 50–100 mL of 20 % sorbitol either orally or by retention enema (50 g of Kayexalate)

For *moderate* elevation *(6–7 mEq/L),* shift potassium intracellularly with the following:

1. Sodium bicarbonate—50 mEq IV over 5 min (sodium bicarbonate alone is less effective than glucose plus insulin or nebulised albuterol, particularly for the treatment of patients with renal failure; it is best used in conjunction with these medications) [67, 68]
2. Glucose plus insulin—mix 50 g glucose and 10 U regular insulin and give IV over 15–30 min
3. Nebulised albuterol 10–20 mg nebulised over 15 min

For *severe* elevation *(>7 mEq/L* with toxic ECG changes), you need to shift potassium into the cells and eliminate potassium from the body. Therapies that shift potassium will act rapidly, but they are temporary; if the serum potassium rebounds, you may need to repeat those therapies. In order of priority, treatment includes the following:

* *Shift potassium into cells:*
    1. Calcium chloride (10 %): 500–1000 mg (5–10 mL) IV over 2–5 min to reduce the effects of potassium at the myocardial cell membrane (lowers risk of VF)
    2. Sodium bicarbonate: 50 mEq IV over 5 min (may be less effective for patients with end-stage renal disease)
    3. Glucose plus insulin: mix 25 g (50 mL of D50) glucose and 10 U regular insulin and give IV over 15–30 min

    4. Nebulised albuterol: 10–20 mg nebulised over 15 min
- *Promote potassium excretion:*
    5. Diuresis (furosemide 40–80 mg IV)
    6. Kayexalate enema: 15–50 g plus sorbitol PO or per rectum
    7. Dialysis

Treatment of Hypokalaemia

Treatment of hypokalaemia focuses on parenteral and oral potassium supplementation as well as identification and treatment of the source of the electrolyte abnormality. IV administration of potassium is indicated when arrhythmias are present or hypokalaemia is *severe (<2.5 mEq/L)*. Gradual correction of hypokalaemia is preferable to rapid correction unless the patient is clinically unstable. Acute potassium administration may be empirical in emergent conditions. When indicated, maximum IV K^+ replacement should be 10–20 mEq/h with continuous ECG monitoring during infusion. Central or peripheral IV sites may be used. A more concentrated solution of potassium may be infused if a central line is used, but the catheter tip should not extend into the right atrium.

If cardiac arrest from hypokalaemia is imminent (i.e. malignant ventricular arrhythmias), rapid replacement of potassium is required. Give an initial infusion of 10 mEq IV over 5 min; repeat once if needed. In the patient's chart, document that rapid infusion is intentional in response to life-threatening hypokalaemia. Once the patient is stabilised, reduce the infusion to continue potassium replacement more gradually. Estimates of total body deficit of potassium range from 150 to 400 mEq for every 1 mEq decrease in serum potassium. The lower range of the estimate would be appropriate for an elderly woman with low muscle mass and the higher range for a young, muscular man.

Treatment of Hypermagnesaemia

Hypermagnesaemia is treated with administration of *calcium*, which removes magnesium from serum. Cardiorespiratory support may be needed until magnesium levels are reduced. It is important to eliminate sources of ongoing magnesium intake. Administration of 10 % solution of calcium chloride (5–10 mL [500–1000 mg] IV) will often correct lethal arrhythmias. This dose may be repeated if needed. Dialysis is the treatment of choice for hypermagnesaemia. Until that can be done, if renal function is normal and cardiovascular function adequate, IV saline dieresis (IV normal saline and furosemide) can be used to increase renal excretion of magnesium until dialysis can be performed. However, this diuresis can also increase calcium excretion; the development of hypocalcaemia will deteriorate signs and symptoms of hypermagnesaemia.

Treatment of Hypomagnesaemia

Treatment of hypomagnesaemia depends on its severity and the patient's clinical status. For severe or symptomatic hypomagnesaemia, administer 1–2 g IV MgSO4 over 5–60 min. For torsades de pointes with cardiac arrest, give 1–2 g of MgSO4 IV pushed over 5–20 min. If torsades de pointes is intermittent and not associated with arrest, administer the magnesium over 5–60 min IV. If seizures are present, administer 2 g IV MgSO4 over 10 min. Calcium gluconate administration (1 g) is usually appropriate because most patients with hypomagnesaemia are also hypocalcaemic [69]. Replace magnesium cautiously in patients with renal insufficiency because there is a real danger of causing life-threatening hypermagnesaemia.

Treatment of Hypercalcaemia

If hypercalcaemia is due to malignancy, careful consideration of the patient's prognosis and wishes is needed. Therapy for hypercalcaemia is generally instituted based on clinical signs more than absolute serum levels, although empiric therapy is often started at levels of 12 mg/dL even in the asymptomatic patient. In patients with hypoalbuminaemia, measured serum calcium levels may mask significant elevations in free ionised extracellular calcium. Treatment is instituted at a level *>15 mg/dL* regardless of symptoms. Immediate therapy is directed at promoting calcium excretion in the urine. The mainstays of treatment are intravenous volume repletion and bisphosphonate agents that inhibit osteoclastic bone resorption. This is accomplished in patients with adequate cardiovascular and renal function with infusion of 0.9 % saline at 300–500 mL/h until any fluid deficit is replaced and diuresis occurs (urine output 200–300 mL/h). Once adequate rehydration has occurred, the saline infusion rate is reduced to 100–200 mL/h. This diuresis will further reduce serum potassium and magnesium concentrations, which may increase the arrhythmogenic potential of the hypercalcaemia. Thus, potassium and magnesium concentrations should be closely monitored and maintained. Hemodialysis is the treatment of choice to rapidly decrease serum calcium in patients with heart failure or renal insufficiency [70]. The use of loop diuretics (furosemide 1 mg/kg IV) to promote calciuresis is often recommended but is problematic in the hypovolemic patient.

Treatment of Hypocalcaemia

Calcium exchange is dependent on concentrations of potassium and magnesium, so treatment depends on replacing all 3 electrolytes.

Treatment of hypocalcaemia requires administration of calcium. Treat acute, symptomatic hypocalcaemia with 10 % calcium gluconate, 90–180 mg of elemental calcium IV over 10 min. Follow this with an IV drip of 540–720 mg of elemental calcium in 500–1000 mL D5W at 0.5–2.0 mg/kg per hour (10–15 mg/kg). Measure serum calcium every 4–6 h. Aim to maintain the total serum calcium concentration between 7 and 9 mg/dL.

Vitamin D and oral calcium supplementation can be administered for chronic hypocalcaemia.

9.1.2.3 When Should Electrolyte Level Be Rechecked?

The studies did not address the frequency and duration of monitoring of patients with ion disturbances; therefore, recommendations regarding ongoing assessment are based on opinion. In the acute management of electrolyte deficiency/excess, the frequency of monitoring depends on the electrolyte level as well as underlying comorbidities. After initial interventions, electrolyte level should be rechecked within *1–2 h*, to ensure effectiveness of the intervention, following which the frequency of monitoring could be reduced. Subsequent monitoring depends on the electrolyte abnormalities and the potential reversibility of the underlying cause.

> We believe the management and treatment of metabolic disorders and ion disturbances that can lead to severe complications, such as life-threatening arrhythmias, should be common knowledge for both the physician working in ED and for the cardiologist. Here, however, we emphasise some peculiarities related to the disorders described that can be particularly useful.

9.2   What Physicians Working in ED Should Know

Profound diarrhoea has the potential to 'waste' large quantities of essential electrolytes, in addition to water and bicarbonate. Without appropriate and timely management, it is possible to develop a highly proarrhythmic situation with metabolic acidosis, increased adrenergic activity, hypokalaemia, hypocalcaemia, hypomagnesaemia and so on. Vomiting can equally result in many of these abnormalities and so in combination with diarrhoea, or when added to other disease states such as DKA, can cause a significant combined cardiac insult. Appropriate identification of these metabolic and fluid balance abnormalities is imperative in order to prevent complications. Thus, regular assessment of hydration, acid-base and electrolyte status is crucial.

Potassium
- Evaluation of serum potassium must consider the effects of changes in serum pH. When serum pH falls, serum potassium rises because potassium shifts from the cellular to the vascular space. When serum pH rises, serum potassium falls because potassium shifts intracellularly. In general, serum K decreases by approximately 0.3 mEq/L for every 0.1 U increase in pH above normal. Effects of pH changes on serum potassium should be anticipated during therapy for hyperkalaemia or hypokalaemia and during any therapy that may cause changes in serum pH (e.g. treatment of diabetic ketoacidosis). Correction of an alkalotic pH will produce an increase in serum potassium even without administration of additional potassium. If serum potassium is 'normal' in the face of acidosis, a fall in serum potassium should be anticipated when the acidosis is corrected, and potassium administration should be planned.
- Hypokalaemia exacerbates digitalis toxicity. Thus, hypokalaemia should be avoided or treated promptly in patients receiving digitalis derivatives.
- The ECG correlates of hypokalaemia can be confused with myocardial ischemia. In addition, it can be difficult to differentiate a U wave from a peaked T wave that is present in hyperkalaemia.
- The use of a beta-agonist appeared to be effective in rapid reduction of hyperkalaemia: salbutamol is effective when given intravenously, in a nebulised form and

as a multi-dose inhaler. IV insulin and glucose is effective and has a rapid onset of action. The evidence for the use of bicarbonate in hyperkalaemia is equivocal, and it is not recommended as monotherapy. If used in conjunction with other treatments, the possible effects on pH and extracellular volume must be carefully considered in the assessment of the risk-benefit ratio for an individual patient.

Combining insulin-glucose with salbutamol (albuterol) probably leads to greater reductions in serum potassium than either alone. In animal and human studies, IV calcium stabilises membranes and reduces the arrhythmic threshold. Though no randomised evidence exists to support its use, it is recommended that calcium chloride be given in the presence of ECG changes or arrhythmia and repeated as needed.

Magnesium
- Abnormalities in magnesium, potassium and pH must be corrected simultaneously.
- Untreated hypomagnesaemia will make hypocalcaemia refractory to therapy.

Calcium
- The concentration of ionised calcium is pH dependent. Alkalosis increases the binding of calcium to albumin and thus reduces ionised calcium. Conversely, the development of acidosis will produce an increase in the ionised calcium level.
- In the presence of hypoalbuminaemia, although total calcium level may be low, the ionised calcium level may be normal.
- Calcium antagonises the effects of both potassium and magnesium at the cell membrane. Therefore, it is extremely useful for treating the effects of hyperkalaemia and hypermagnesaemia.
- Calcium may also be lowered by drugs that reduce bone resorption (e.g. calcitonin, glucocorticoids).

9.3   What Cardiologists Should Know

A diverse array of metabolic disorders is known to precipitate arrhythmia, though their individual proarrhythmic effects can be simplified by considering broad unifying pathophysiological mechanisms.

Metabolic disturbance mediates re-entry because regions of physiologically and pathological conduction (accelerated myocyte repolarisation or reduced myocardial conduction velocity) are both present, although anatomical substrates can interact and so produce complex disturbances of myocardial excitation and conduction.

Acidosis is proarrhythmic through promoting re-entry and triggered activity [71]. It is notable that re-entry on a much larger scale is the cause of certain supraventricular tachycardia, for example, atrioventricular re-entry tachycardia in the Wolff-Parkinson-White syndrome. Metabolic derangement can alter the conduction properties of the abnormal anatomic pathways in these disorders, promoting re-entry and/or augmenting the maximum heart rate supported by the circuit. More complex re-entry is also a contributory factor to other arrhythmias witnessed in critically ill patients, such as atrial fibrillation and VT. After-depolarisation, or triggered activity, is the other major mechanism through which electrolyte disturbance encourages arrhythmias.

This process may be repeated resulting in tachycardia, and it is through this mechanism in which polymorphic VT, or torsades de pointes, develops. Delayed after-depolarisations are less relevant to proarrhythmia in the context of pure metabolic disarray, though in certain circumstances remain relevant. The classical example is arrhythmia due to digoxin toxicity which is aggravated by hypokalaemia and hypercalcaemia. Catecholamine excess and myocardial ischaemia are also important, and relatively common, precipitants in patients with metabolic disarray.

Potassium
- Interestingly, bypass tracts are more sensitive to delayed conduction from potassium elevation, which can result in the normalisation of the ECG and loss of the delta wave in patients with Wolff-Parkinson-White syndrome.
- With extremely high serum potassium levels, a markedly prolonged and wide QRS complex can fuse with the T wave, producing a slurred, 'sine-wave' appearance on the ECG. This finding is a pre-terminal event unless treatment is initiated immediately. The fatal event is either asystole, as there is complete block in ventricular conduction, or ventricular fibrillation.
- Hyperkalaemia can induce a Brugada-like pattern in the ECG [72]. This usually occurs in critically ill patient with significant hyperkalaemia (serum potassium >7.0 mmol/L) and is associated with pseudo-right bundle branch block and persistent coved ST segment elevation in at least two precordial leads. Prompt recognition of this ECG entity will enable clinicians to identify severe hyperkalaemia, which may result in high mortality.
- The effect of hyperkalaemia on QRS morphology of ventricular paced beats has also been studied [73]: hyperkalaemia is the most common electrolyte abnormality to cause loss of capture. In patients with pacemakers, hyperkalaemia causes two important clinical abnormalities: [1] widening of the paced QRS complex (and paced P wave) on the basis of delayed myocardial conduction; when the K level exceeds 7 mEq/L, the intraventricular conduction velocity is usually decreased and the paced QRS complex widens, [2] and increased atrial and ventricular pacing thresholds with or without increased latency.
- In patients with cardiac resynchronisation therapy, the hyperkalaemia can result in a loss of capture and/or sensing failure of even only one of the two ventricular electrodes, leading to a biventricular activation failure.
- Several cardiac and non-cardiac drugs are known to suppress the HERG K+ channel and hence the IK and, especially in the presence of hypokalaemia, can result in prolonged action potential duration and QT interval, early after-depolarisations and torsades de pointes.

- Hyperkalaemia is a common disorder that can be fatal if unrecognised or untreated. Insulin administered intravenously has the fastest onset of action and is very effective in reducing serum potassium. β2-Adrenergic agonists are as effective as insulin for lowering serum potassium and have a longer duration of action. The combination of β2-agonists and insulin is more effective than either treatment alone. The use of intravenously administered sodium bicarbonate for the management of acute hyperkalaemia is supported only by studies with weak and equivocal results [74] .
- Changes in pH inversely affect serum potassium. Acidosis (low pH) leads to an extracellular shift of potassium, thus raising serum potassium. Conversely, high pH (alkalosis) shifts potassium back into the cell, lowering serum potassium. Metabolic alterations such as alkalosis, hypernatraemia or hypercalcaemia can antagonise the transmembrane effects of hyperkalaemia and result in the blunting of the ECG changes associated with elevated potassium levels.
- Hyperkalaemia inhibits glycoside binding to (Na+, K+) ATPase, decreases the inotropic effect of digitalis and suppresses digitalis-induced ectopic rhythms. Alternatively, hypokalaemia increases glycoside binding to (Na+, K+) ATPase, decreases the rate of digoxin elimination and potentiates the toxic effects of digitalis.

Magnesium
- Low potassium in combination with low magnesium is a risk factor for severe arrhythmias.
- It is well known that both supraventricular and ventricular dysrhythmias can be potentiated if not directly caused by hypomagnesaemia.
- Magnesium has been shown to be efficacious in the management of atrial tachy-dysrhythmias although there is no correlation between rhythm conversion and plasma concentration.
- Magnesium sulphate is considered first-line therapy by the American Heart Association ACLS Guidelines for torsades de pointes.

Calcium
- The combination of hyperkalaemia and hypocalcaemia has a cumulative effect on the atrioventricular and intraventricular conduction delay and facilitates the development of VF. Hypercalcaemia, through its membrane-stabilising effect, counteracts the effects of hyperkalaemia on AV and intraventricular conduction and averts the development of VF.
- Half of all calcium in the extracellular fluid is bound to albumin; the other half is in the biologically active, ionised form. The ionised form is most active. The serum ionised calcium level must be evaluated in light of serum pH and serum albumin.
- Hypocalcaemia can exacerbate digitalis toxicity Table 9.1.

Table 9.1 Ion disturbances: etiology, diagnosis and treatment

Ione	Disorders	Aetiology	Signs	EKG changes	Treatment
K+	Hyperkalaemia mild (5–6 mEq/L)	Drugs End-stage renal disease	Weakness Ascending paralysis Respiratory failure	Flattened P waves Prolonged PR interval	1. Furosemide 1 mg/kg IV slowly 2. Kayexalate 15–30 g in 50–100 mL of 20 % sorbitol
	Hyperkalaemia moderate (6–7 mEq/L)	Rhabdomyolysis Metabolic acidosis Pseudohyperkalaemia Hemolysis Tumour lysis syndrome		Widened QRS complex Deepened S waves Merging of S and T waves	1. Sodium bicarbonate—50 mEq IV over 5 min 2. Glucose plus insulin—mix 50 g glucose and 10 U regular insulin and give IV over 15–30 min 3. Nebulised albuterol 10–20 mg nebulised over 15 min
	Hyperkalaemia severe (>7 mEq/L)	Diet Hypoaldosteronism (Addison disease, hyporeninemia) Type 4 renal tubular acidosis Hyperkalaemic periodic paralysis		Sine-wave pattern Idioventricular rhythm Asystolic cardiac arrest	1. Calcium chloride (10 %): 500–1000 mg (5–10 mL) IV over 2–5 min 2. Sodium bicarbonate: 50 mEq IV over 5 min 3. Glucose plus insulin: mix 25 g (50 mL of D50) glucose and 10 U regular insulin and give IV over 15–30 min 4. Nebulised albuterol: 10–20 mg nebulised over 15 min 5. Furosemide 40–80 mg IV) 6. Kayexalate enema: 15–50 g plus sorbitol PO or per rectum 7. Dialysis
	Hypokalaemia mild (3.5–2.5 mEq/L)	Diarrhoea, Laxatives	Weakness Fatigue Paralysis Respiratory difficulty Constipation Paralytic ileus Leg cramps	U waves T wave flattening	Gradual correction of hypokalaemia is preferable to rapid correction
	Hypokalaemia severe (<2.5 mEq/L)	Hyperaldosteronism Hyperglycaemia Potassium depleting Diuretics Carbenicillin, sodium penicillin, amphotericin B Intracellular shift (alkalosis or a rise in pH) Malnutrition		Ventricular arrhythmias –Pulseless electrical activity (PEA) Asystole	1. Maximum IV K replacement should be 10 to 20 mEq/h 2. Infusion of 10 mEq IV over 5 min (if cardiac arrest)

(continued)

Table 9.1 (continued)

Ione	Disorders	Aetiology	Signs	EKG changes	Treatment
Mg+	*Hypermagnesaemia* (>2.2 mEq/L)	Renal failure Overuse of mg+ Use of laxatives/antacids containing mg+	Areflexia Muscular weakness Paralysis Ataxia Drowsiness Confusion Respiratory failure Nausea Vomiting Hypotension Hypoventilation	Increased PR and QT Increased QRS Decrease P wave voltage Degree of T wave peaking Complete AV block Asystole	1. 10 % solution of calcium chloride (5–10 mL [500–1000 mg] IV) 2. Dialysis 3. Furosemide [1 mEq/kg]
	Hypomagnesaemia (<1.3 mEq/L)	Bowel resection Pancreatitis Diarrhoea Renal disease Diuretics Pentamidine Gentamicin Digoxin Alcohol Hypothermia Hypercalcaemia Diabetic ketoacidosis Hyperthyroidism Hypothyroidism Phosphate deficiency Burns Sepsis	Seizures Mental status changes Dysrhythmias Vasospasm Hypokalaemia Hypocalcaemia Bronchospasm Muscle weakness	Prolonged QT and PR intervals ST segment depression T wave inversion Flattening P waves Widening of QRS Torsades de pointes VF	1. 1–2 g IV MgSO4 over 5–60 min 2. For torsades de pointes 1 to 2 g of MgSO4 IV over 5–20 min

Ca++	*Hypercalcaemia* > 10.5 mEq/L (or > 4.8 mg/dL ionised calcium)	Hyperparathyroidism Malignancy	Fatigue Lethargy Motor weakness Anorexia Nausea Constipation Abdominal pain Diuresis Hallucinations Disorientation Hypotonicity	Shortened QT interval Prolonged PR and QRS intervals Increased QRS voltage T wave flattening and widening Notching of QRS AV block	1. 0.9 % saline at 300 to 500 mL/h 2. Hemodialysis 3. Chelating agents 4. Furosemide 5. Calcitonin, glucocorticoids
	Hypocalcaemia < 8.5 mg/dL (or < 4.2 mg/dL ionised calcium)	Toxic shock Abnormalities in serum magnesium Tumour lysis syndrome	Neuromuscular irritability Carpal-pedal spasm –Tetany Laryngospasm Paraesthesias of the extremities and face Muscle cramps Hyperreflexia Positive Chvostek and Trousseau signs	QT interval prolongation Terminal T wave inversion Heart blocks Ventricular fibrillation	1. 10 % calcium gluconate, 90–180 mg of calcium IV over 10 min 2. IV drip of 540–720 mg of elemental calcium in 500–1000 mL D_5W at 0.5–2.0 mg/kg per hour (10–15 mg/kg)

Bibliography

1. El-Sherif N, Turitto G. Electrolyte disorders and arrhythmogenesis. Cardiol J. 2011;18:233–45.
2. Kraft MD, Btaiche IF, Sacks GS, et al. Treatment of electrolyte disorders in adult patients in the intensive care unit. Am J Health Syst Pharm. 2005;62:1663–82.
3. Task FM, Zipes DP, Camm AJ, et al. ACC/AHA/ESC 2006 guidelines for management of patients with ventricular arrhythmias and the prevention of sudden cardiac death – executive summary: A report of the American College of Cardiology/American Heart Association Task Force and the European Society of Cardiology Committee for Practice Guidelines (Writing Committee to Develop Guidelines for Management of Patients with Ventricular Arrhythmias and the Prevention of Sudden Cardiac Death). Developed in collaboration with the European Heart Rhythm Association and the Heart Rhythm Society. Eur Heart J. 2006;27:2099–140.
4. Whalley DW, Wendt DJ, Grant AO. Electrophysiologic effects of acute ischemia and reperfusion and their role in the genesis of cardiac arrhythmias. In: Podrid PJ, Kowey PR, editors. Cardiac arrhythmia: mechanisms, diagnosis, and management. Baltimore: Williams & Wilkins; 1995. p. 109–30.
5. Ramaswamy K, Hamdan MH. Ischemia, metabolic disturbances, and arrhythmogenesis: mechanisms and management. Crit Care Med. 2000;28(Suppl):N151–7.
6. Nesher G, Zion MM. Recurrent ventricular tachycardia in hypothyroidism report of a case and review of the literature. Cardiology. 1988;75:301–6.
7. Osborn LA, Skipper B, Arellano I, et al. Results of resting and ambulatory electrocardiograms in patients with hypothyroidism and after return to euthyroid status. Heart Dis. 1999;1:8–11.
8. Singh AK, Nguyen PN. Refractory ventricular tachycardia following aortic valve replacement complicated by unsuspected pheochromocytoma. Thorac Cardiovasc Surg. 1993;41:372–3.
9. Michaels RD, Hays JH, O'Brian JT, et al. Pheochromocytoma associated ventricular tachycardia blocked with atenolol. J Endocrinol Invest. 1990;13:943–7.
10. Shimizu K, Miura Y, Meguro Y, et al. QT prolongation with torsades de pointes in pheochromocytoma. Am Heart J. 1992;124:235–9.
11. Viskin S, Fish R, Roth A, et al. Clinical problem-solving. QT or not QT? N Engl J Med. 2000;343:352–6.
12. Colao A. Are patients with acromegaly at high risk for dysrhythmias? Clin Endocrinol (Oxf). 2001;55:305–6.
13. Kahaly G, Olshausen KV, Mohr-Kahaly S, et al. Arrhythmia profile in acromegaly. Eur Heart J. 1992;13:51–6.
14. Colao A, Ferone D, Marzullo P, et al. Long-term effects of depot long-acting somatostatin analog octreotide on hormone levels and tumor mass in acromegaly. J Clin Endocrinol Metab. 2001;86:2779–86.
15. Minniti G, Moroni C, Jaffrain-Rea ML, et al. Marked improvement in cardiovascular function after successful transsphenoidal surgery in acromegalic patients. Clin Endocrinol (Oxf). 2001;55:307–13.
16. Suyama K, Uchida D, Tanaka T, et al. Octreotide improved ventricular arrhythmia in an acromegalic patient. Endocr J. 2000;47(Suppl):S73–5.
17. Lombardi G, Colao A, Marzullo P, et al. Improvement of left ventricular hypertrophy and arrhythmias after lanreotide-induced GH and IGF-I decrease in acromegaly. A prospective multi-center study. J Endocrinol Invest. 2002;25:971–6.
18. Colao A, Marzullo P, Cuocolo A, et al. Reversal of acromegalic cardiomyopathy in young but not in middle-aged patients after 12 months of treatment with the depot long-acting somatostatin analogue octreotide. Clin Endocrinol (Oxf). 2003;58:169–76.
19. Izumi C, Inoko M, Kitaguchi S, et al. Polymorphic ventricular tachycardia in a patient with adrenal insufficiency and hypothyroidism. Jpn Circ J. 1998;62:543–5.
20. Abdo A, Bebb RA, Wilkins GE. Ventricular fibrillation: an extreme presentation of primary hyperaldosteronism. Can J Cardiol. 1999;15:347–8; 549.

21. Chang CJ, Chen SA, Tai CT, et al. Ventricular tachycardia in a patient with primary hyperpara-thyroidism. Pacing Clin Electrophysiol. 2000;23:534–7.
22. Wallace TM, Matthews DR. Recent advances in the monitoring and management of diabetic ketoacidosis. QJM. 2004;97:773–80.
23. Harrower C. The value of continuous ECG monitoring during treatment of diabetic ketoacidosis. A computer study. Acta Diabetol Lat. 1975;15:88–94.
24. American Heart Association. Guidelines for cardiopulmonary resuscitation and emergency cardiovascular care: life-threatening electrolyte abnormalities. Circulation. 2005;112:IV-121–5.
25. Diercks DB, Shumaik GM, Harrigan RA, Brady WJ, Chan TC. Electrocardiographic manifestations: electrolyte abnormalities. J Emerg Med. 2004;27:153–60.
26. Brobst D. Review of the pathophysiology of alterations in potassium homeostasis. J Am Vet Med Assoc. 1986;188:1019–25.
27. Brown RS. Potassium homeostasis and clinical implications. Am J Med. 1984;77:3–10.
28. Yu AS. Atypical electrocardiographic changes in severe hyperkalemia. Am J Cardiol. 1990;77:906–8.
29. Martinez-Vea A, Bardaji A, Garcia C, Oliver JA. Severe hyperkalemia with minimal electrocardiographic manifestations: a report of seven cases. J Electrocardiol. 1999;32:45–9.
30. Moore ML, Bailey RR. Hyperkalaemia in patients in hospital. N Z Med J. 1989;102:557–8.
31. Stevens MS, Dunlay RW. Hyperkalemia in hospitalized patients. Int Urol Nephrol. 2000;32:177–80.
32. Paice B, Gray JM, McBride D, et al. Hyperkalaemia in patients in hospital. Br Med J (Clin Res Ed). 1983;286:1189–92.
33. Shemer J, Modan M, Ezra D, et al. Incidence of hyperkalemia in hospitalized patients. Isr J Med Sci. 1983;19:659–61.
34. Surawicz B. Relationship between electrocardiogram and electrolytes. Am Heart J. 1967;73:814–34.
35. Freeman K, Feldman JA, Mitchell P, et al. Effects of presentation and electrocardiogram on time to treatment of hyperkalemia. Acad Emerg Med. 2008;15:239–49.
36. Fisch C. Relation of electrolyte disturbances to cardiac arrhythmias. Circulation. 1973;47:408–19.
37. Jackson MA, Lodwick R, Hutchinson SG. Hyperkalaemic cardiac arrest successfully treated with peritoneal dialysis. BMJ. 1996;312:1289–90.
38. Voelckel W, Kroesen G. Unexpected return of cardiac action after termination of cardiopulmonary resuscitation. Resuscitation. 1996;32:27–9.
39. Niemann JT, Cairns CB. Hyperkalemia and ionized hypocalcemia during cardiac arrest and resuscitation: possible culprits for postcountershock arrhythmias? Ann Emerg Med. 1999;34:1–7.
40. Slovis C, Jenkins R. Conditions not primarily affecting the heart. BMJ. 2002;324:1320–3.
41. Mattu A, Brady WJ, Robinson DA. Electrocardiographic manifestations of hyperkalemia. Am J Emerg Med. 2000;18:721–6.
42. Webster A, Brady W, Morris F. Recognising signs of danger: EKG changes resulting from an abnormal serum potassium concentration. Emerg Med J. 2002;19:74–7.
43. Ettinger PO, Regan TJ, Oldewurtel HA. Hyperkalemia, cardiac conduction and the electrocardiogram: a review. Am Heart J. 1974;88:360–71.
44. Levine HD, Wanzer SH, Merrill JP. Dialyzable currents of injury in potassium intoxication resembling acute myocardial infarction or pericarditis. Circulation. 1956;13:29–36.
45. Paice BJ, Paterson KR, Onyanga-Omara F, et al. Record linkage study of hypokalemia in hospitalized patients. Postgrad Med J. 1986;62:187–91.
46. Schulman M, Narins RG. Hypokalemia and cardiovascular disease. Am J Cardiol. 1990;65:4E–9.
47. Thompson RG, Gobb LA. Hypokalemia after resuscitation out-of-hospital ventricular fibrillation. JAMA. 1982;248:2860–3.
48. Surawicz B, Braun HA, Crum WB, et al. Quantitative analysis of the electrocardiographic pattern of hypopotassemia. Circulation. 1957;16:750–63.

49. Surawicz B. Electrolytes and the electrocardiogram. Postgrad Med. 1974;55:123–9.
50. Yan GX, Lankipalli RS, Burke JK, Musco S, Kowey PR. Ventricular repolarization components of the electrocardiogram: cellular basis and clinical significance. J Am Coll Cardiol. 2003;42:401.
51. Agus ZS, Wasserstein A, Goldfarb S. Disorders of calcium and magnesium homeostasis. Am J Med. 1982;72:473–9.
52. Dyckner T, Wester PO. Relation between potassium, magnesium and cardiac arrhythmias. Acta Med Scand Suppl. 1981;647:163–9.
53. Navarro-Gonzalez JF. Magnesium in dialysis patients: serum levels and clinical implications. Clin Nephrol. 1998;49:373–8.
54. Fiset C, Kargacin ME, Kondo CS, Lester WM, Duff HJ. Hypomagnesemia: characterization of a model of sudden cardiac death. J Am Coll Cardiol. 1996;27:1771–6.
55. Leier CV, Dei Cas L, Metra M. Clinical relevance and management of the major electrolyte abnormalities in congestive heart failure: hyponatremia, hypokalemia, and hypomagnesemia. Am Heart J. 1994;128:564–74.
56. Bushinsky DA, Monk RD. Electrolyte quintet: calcium. Lancet. 1998;352:306–11.
57. Barri YM, Knochel JP. Hypercalcemia and electrolyte disturbances in malignancy. Hematol Oncol Clin North Am. 1996;10:775–90.
58. Aldinger KA, Samaan NA. Hypokalemia with hypercalcemia: prevalence and significance in treatment. Ann Intern Med. 1977;87:571–3.
59. Ziegler R. Hypercalcemic crisis. J Am Soc Nephrol. 2001;12 Suppl 17:S3–9.
60. Carlstedt F, Lind L. Hypocalcemic syndromes. Crit Care Clin. 2001;17:139–53.
61. Campistol JM, Almirall J, Montoliu J, Revert L. Electrographic alterations induced by hyperkalaemia simulating acute myocardial infarction. Nephrol Dial Transplant. 1989;4:233–5.
62. Forsythe SM, Schmidt GA. Sodium bicarbonate for the treatment of lactic acidosis. Chest. 2000;117:260–7.
63. Viallon AM, Zeni FM, Lafond PM, et al. Does bicarbonate therapy improve the management of severe diabetic ketoacidosis? Crit Care Med. 1999;27:2690–3.
64. Committee M, Blomstrom-Lundqvist C, Scheinman MM, et al. ACC/AHA/ESC guidelines for the management of patients with supraventricular arrhythmias-executive summary: A Report of the American College of Cardiology/American Heart Association Task Force on Practice Guidelines and the European Society of Cardiology Committee for Practice Guidelines (Writing Committee to Develop Guidelines for the Management of Patients With Supraventricular Arrhythmias) Developed in collaboration with NASPE-Heart Rhythm Society. Eur Heart J. 2003;24:1857–97.
65. Friedman P, Stevenson W. Proarrhythmia. Am J Cardiol. 1998;82:50N–8.
66. Weisberg LS. Management of severe hyperkalemia. Crit Care Med. 2008;36:3246–51.
67. Ngugi NN, McLigeyo SO, Kayima JK. Treatment of hyperkalaemia by altering the transcellular gradient in patients with renal failure: effect of various therapeutic approaches. East Afr Med J. 1997;74:503–9.
68. Allon M, Shanklin N. Effect of bicarbonate administration on plasma potassium in dialysis patients: interactions with insulin and albuterol. Am J Kidney Dis. 1996;28:508–14.
69. al-Ghamdi SM, Cameron EC, Sutton RA. Magnesium deficiency: pathophysiologic and clinical overview [see comments]. Am J Kidney Dis. 1994;24:737–52.
70. Edelson GW, Kleerekoper M. Hypercalcemic crisis. Med Clin North Am. 1995;79:79–92.
71. Orchard CH, Cingolani HE. Acidosis and arrhythmias in cardiac muscle. Cardiovasc Res. 1994;28:1312–9.
72. Littmann L, Monroe MH, Taylor 3rd L, Brearley Jr WD. The hyperkalemic Brugada sign. J Electrocardiol. 2007;40:53–9.
73. Barold SS, Leonelli F, Herweg B. Hyperkalemia during cardiac pacing. Pacing Clin Electrophysiol. 2007;30:1–3.
74. Elliott MJ, Ronksley PE, Catherine M, Ahmed SB, Hemmelgarn BR. Management of patients with acute hyperkalemia. CMAJ. 2010;10:182–15.

Cardiac Arrhythmias in Drug Abuse and Intoxication

10

Laura Vitali-Serdoz, Francesco Furlanello, and Ilaria Puggia

10.1 Focusing on the Issue

Cardiac arrhythmias are common in acute intoxication, although epidemiological data are often restricted to specific substances. A 10 % incidence of cardiac arrhythmias during acute intoxication has been reported by a referral poison center in Germany that analyzed the data of 91,285 patients referred between 1995 and 2003 using the inquiries of physicians and paramedics [1].

A large amount of substances and their association can lead to worsening of preclinical or active cardiovascular diseases and, on occasion, to ex-novo cardiovascular diseases or arrhythmic manifestations. Negative cardiovascular effects are mainly caused by the pharmacokinetics of substances, in particular if drugs are administered or abused in combination, or in cases of concomitant metabolic, renal, or liver diseases; moreover, negative effects can be the result of pharmacodynamics, as in the presence of an interaction between a not otherwise toxic substance and an altered morphofunctional cardiac substrate (e.g., long QT or Brugada syndrome).

L. Vitali-Serdoz (✉)
Klinikum Fürth, Clinic for Heart and
Lung Disease, Electrophysiology Section, Fürth, Germany
e-mail: lavise@gmail.com

F. Furlanello
Humanitas Research Hospital, Rozzano Milano Gavazzeni
Bergamo Cardiac Arrhythmias and Electrophysiology II,
Villa Bianca Hospital, Trento, Italy

I. Puggia
Cardiovascular Department, Ospedali Riuniti and University of Trieste, Trieste, Italy

© Springer International Publishing Switzerland 2016
M. Zecchin, G. Sinagra (eds.), *The Arrhythmic Patient in the Emergency Department: A Practical Guide for Cardiologists and Emergency Physicians*,
DOI 10.1007/978-3-319-24328-3_10

10.2 What Physicians Working in Emergency Departments Should Know

The management of patients with a certain diagnosis or at high risk for "poisoning" or "drug abuse" should be oriented toward the acute handling of symptoms of intoxication and support of hemodynamics (e.g., intubation and respiratory support, electrolyte substitution and hydration, and temporary pacing in the case of bradycardia).

Physicians working in the emergency department (ED) should be aware that people using or abusing illicit drugs are often prone to mix different substances, alcohol being the most abused and coabused substance. Cannabis is the most frequently used illicit drug, followed by cocaine, ecstasy, and amphetamines [2]. Physicians in the ED should be familiar with the telephone number of the local poison control center as well as internal protocols and resources.

When deciding the therapeutic strategy, the medical history of the patient plays a pivotal role, and it is important to follow a systematic approach, starting with the following:

- Habitual medications
- Coexisting diseases
- Which substance or mix was taken, and when
- If a mix of substances was taken, which was the sequela
- Way of substance abuse: pills, sublingual, intravenous, inhalation

It is then important to initiate a treatment as soon as possible in order to achieve a stabilization:

- Cardiopulmonary support including fluids, direct current shock if hemodynamically unstable arrhythmia, or temporary pacing if bradycardia
- Gastrointestinal decontamination of an ingested drug
- Administration of an antidote if available
- Correction of acid–base and electrolyte alterations

10.3 What Physicians Working in the ED and Cardiologists Should Know

In order to offer a pragmatic approach to the management of patients presenting with arrhythmias associated with drug abuse and intoxication, this section focuses firstly on recreational drugs and secondly on the most common prescription drugs.

10.3.1 Recreational Drugs

The use and abuse of recreational drugs is increasing, and every year new "designer drugs" appear on the recreational drug market, such as the novel class of cathinone derivatives, often proposed as "legal highs" by categorizing them as odorizers, stain removers, potpourri, or most recently the notorious "bath salts" [3].

An updated list of many recreational drugs can be easily found by consulting the web site of the World Anti-Doping Agency [4] (WADA list 2015, updated yearly; www.wada-ama.org). This list comprises all those substances abused by the general population and in particular by athletes with ergogenic scope during their lifetime. Many of these drugs can induce cardiovascular effects, particularly arrhythmias, during short-, mid-, and long-term use [5–8].

10.3.1.1 Stimulants

The heterogeneous group of stimulants includes many classes of drugs, widely used to obtain a performance enhancement, a raise in aggressiveness and competitiveness levels, and a reduction of fatigue perception, or simply for "recreational" purposes.

Among stimulants, amphetamines also are widely used for weight-loss regimens [9–11]. Ephedrine and other similar alkaloids are also contained in the herbal product ephedra, marketed as dietary supplement [12, 13].

The amphetamines are the chemical basis of many designer drugs usually sold as "club drugs": methylenedioxymethamphetamine (MDA) is well known as the "love pill," and 3,4-methylenedioxymethamphetamine (MDMA or Ecstasy) is commonly available under confounding names such as "clarity" or "lover's speed," but many chemical variants are commonly abused. The tablets can contain between 50 and 200 mg, and the toxic effects can be manifest starting from a dose of 50 mg [14, 15].

This class of stimulants (amphetamine or ephedrine derivatives) acts through the release of noradrenaline, dopamine, and serotonin. The symptoms of patients presenting in the ED can include sympathomimetic effects such as arterial hypertension, hyperthermia, mydriasis, dry mouth, and tachycardia. Commonly the patients also present with hyperactivity reactions such as logorrhea, restless syndrome, anxiety, tremors, myoclonus and coma.

Regarding the arrhythmias, patients present commonly with sinus or atrial tachycardia, although atrial flutter, atrial fibrillation, supraventricular reentrant tachycardia, and ventricular tachycardia have also been reported. Re-entry arrhythmias may be due to adrenergic activity during myocardial refractory periods [16, 17]. These patients should be treated with intravenous saline volumes, electrolyte substitution, and a β-blocker can be used through a slow intravenous injection for the management of tachycardia and hypertension.

Several cases of cardiac arrest and sudden death in users were reported to be associated with coronary artery disease, cardiomyopathy and myocarditis, and others with direct myocyte toxicity [14, 16]. In patients with Wolff-Parkinson-White (WPW) syndrome, stimulants can induce rapid atrial fibrillation and ventricular fibrillation [18], increasing atrial and ventricular excitability and shortening accessory pathway refractoriness.

Particular attention should be paid to young patients intoxicated with Ecstasy after physically extreme activity (e.g., "rave parties" or athletes after competitions) presenting with a "serotonin syndrome": the combination of central effects (i.e., hyperthermia) and severe dehydration and electrolyte disorders can lead to malignant arrhythmias whose management must combine arrhythmia therapy (cardioversion or β-blocker) with cooling, rehydration, and electrolyte replacement.

Physicians in the ED should also keep in mind that patients with amphetamine intoxication commonly present with associated rhabdomyolysis.

In recent years patients taking a new class of recreational designer drugs based on cathinones mixed with amphetamine, so-called bath salts, have been admitted to the ED. 3,4-Methylenedioxypyrovalerone (MDPV), 4-methylmethcathinone (4-MMC or mephedrone), and 4-methylephedrone are some examples. In the USA, MDPV seems to be the primary active ingredient in the majority of bath salts; on the other hand, in the European Union mephedrone is more common [19].

Cathinone is a β-ketone amphetamine analogue naturally present in the leaves of the plant *Catha edulis* (also known as *Khat*) [3]. Cathinone acts as a mild stimulant by inhibiting monoamine transporters for dopamine, serotonin, and norepinephrine within the central nervous system, and is internationally regulated.

Patients who have taken MDPV may present in the ED with sinus tachycardia and other arrhythmias including ventricular tachycardia [3]. Many different symptoms have been reported, particularly related to a dopaminergic mechanism that leads to serotonin syndrome. It is important to be aware of the prolonged psychogenic effects, which may last for up to 1 week [20]. Deaths after the use of bath salts have been reported [3].

Among cathinone derivatives, only bupropion is legally approved for medical purposes as an antidepressant medication.

10.3.1.2 Cocaine

Cocaine is an alkaloid derived from a plant, *Erythroxylum coca*. It can be inhaled or smoked, only rarely being injected [21, 22]. On the illicit drugs market it can be found as a salt (hydrochloride or sulfate) or a free Base ("crack"). Indeed, this alkaloid may cause different kinds of focal or re-entry supraventricular and ventricular arrhythmias, such as ectopic beats, atrial fibrillation, atrioventricular node re-entry tachycardia, WPW arrhythmias, and nonsustained and sustained ventricular tachycardia and ventricular fibrillation. Arrhythmias are frequently associated with physical effort, which can induce a sympathomimetic effect synergic with cocaine addiction [23].

Regarding electrocardiographic (ECG) alterations and arrhythmias, experimental animal studies on the effects of cocaine showed prolongation of PR, QT, and QTc intervals, a wider QRS, supraventricular and ventricular ectopic activity, ventricular tachycardia, and ventricular fibrillation [21, 24–26].

Cocaine can lead to cardiac side effects through multiple arrhythmogenic mechanisms:

- Local anesthetic effect with block of both sodium and potassium channels
- Sympathomimetic effect with α- and β-receptor stimulation, and consequent increase in heart rate and atrial and ventricular excitability
- Intracellular calcium overload (afterdepolarization arrhythmias)
- Arrhythmias due to ischemia/reperfusion mechanisms
- Increase in heart rate through vagolytic effect
- Inhibitor of generations and conduction of the action potential, with prolongation of QRS caused by sodium channel-blocking effects [27].

Arrhythmias may be also "secondary" to systemic effects of the drug such as hyperthermia, acidosis, stroke or subarachnoid haemorrhage or in Crack-smokers also to pneumotorax. The ability of cocaine to cause myocardial infarction, frequently with severe complications, is well known [22, 23, 28, 29], with the risk in the first hour after use increasing by up to 24-fold [30].

Myocardial infarction as well as various arrhythmias can occur even after the first administration of cocaine, regardless of dose.

In the ED the patients who have used/abused cocaine may present with many different types of arrhythmias whether in the setting of ischemic/reperfusion events or not. "Chaotic atrial arrhythmia," similar to that observed in severe respiratory insufficiency or acute myocarditis, is considered a typical toxic cocaine-related arrhythmia (Fig. 10.1). Moreover, supraventricular tachycardia, atrial fibrillation, ventricular tachycardia/fibrillation, torsade des pointes due to secondary long QT syndrome frequently related to hERG potassium channel blockade [25, 31], asystole (sporadic reports of asystole treated with emergent cardiac pacing), and cardiac arrest [18] have also been reported. Cocaine-induced wide complex ventricular tachycardia may be considered a typical toxic arrhythmia, frequently caused by high doses of the drug [22], and the treatment is based on administration of sodium bicarbonate [32].

Cocaine can also induce ECG modifications such as a V1–V3 ST elevation (coved type) typical for Brugada syndrome, due to a selective block of myocardial sodium channels in subjects with latent arrhythmic disease [33].

Moreover, patients abusing cocaine also commonly mix it with different substances such as hallucinogens, strychnine ("dead hit"), heroin ("speedball"), and alcohol ("liquid lady"): in case of associated intake of alcohol and cocaine the risk of sudden death has been found to be higher probably because of the additive effects of a metabolite, coca-ethylene, which can block the dopamine reuptake, enhancing the toxic effect of the cocaine used alone [34].

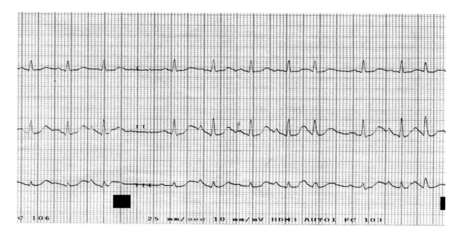

Fig. 10.1 Amateur football player, 17 years old, suspected cocaine intoxication and "chaotic atrial arrhythmia," i.e., sinus rhythm and polymorphic supraventricular ectopic beats

10.3.1.3 Cannabinoids

Many patients can present to the ED after consumption of cannabinoids, including marijuana and hashish, with different arrhythmic disorders: exercise-related sinus tachycardia, atrial fibrillation, paroxysmal supraventricular tachycardia, supraventricular and/or ventricular ectopic beats, and severe ventricular arrhythmias [35, 36], which can be mediated by catecholamines (Fig. 10.2).

The onset of arrhythmias is usually 30 or 60 min after smoking, and the arrhythmic disorders are related to the dose. At low and moderate doses there is an increase in sympathetic activity and a decrease in parasympathetic activity, and patients commonly present with sinus tachycardia, ectopic beats, or paroxysmal supraventricular tachycardia. At higher doses, there is a decrease in sympathetic activity and an increase in parasympathetic activity that can favour atrial fibrillation [37].

10.3.2 Prescription Drugs

Different common prescription drugs can induce arrhythmic complications in cases of involuntary abuse, suicidality, or in case of multiple interactions. Rather than providing an exhaustive list of all possible arrhythmias related to the use or abuse of prescription drugs, this section aims to help physicians working in the ED to get

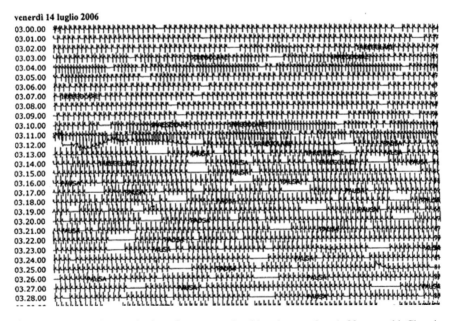

Fig. 10.2 ECG-Holter monitoring of a young male athlete (soccer player), 22 years old. Chronic use of cannabinoids and sporadic use of cocaine. This ECG-Holter tracing taken overnight shows a sick sinus syndrome with sinus arrest, sinus tachycardia, and nonsustained atrial tachycardia

used to a comprehensive attitude on managing not only the arrhythmias but also the whole pathologic affections.

Here, the most common prescription drugs whose abuse or misuse can present with arrhythmias are reviewed.

10.3.2.1 β-Blockers

Abuse of β-blockers can induce bradyarrhythmias with atrio-ventricular blocks of various degrees, sinus bradycardia, junctional and ventricular escape rhythms, bradycardia-dependent ventricular ectopic beats, and asystole, especially in patients with underlying structural and electrical disorders. Among the β-blockers, sotalol is associated with a high rate of cardiac dysrhythmias [1] and related QT prolongation. Other symptoms can be associated as hypotension, syncope, muscular contractions, mydriasis, bronchial obstruction and often hypoglycaemia especially in children.

The doctors in the ER should perform a gastrointestinal decontamination with activated charcoal and a correction of the hypoglicemia and other electrolyte disorders if present. Intravenous dopamine or adrenaline may be necessary, and the cardiologist should prepare a central venous access for a promt temporary pacing if required.

10.3.2.2 Digitalis

Patients presenting in the ED with symptoms of digitalis intoxication, mainly gastrointestinal in nature, such as anorexia, nausea, and vomiting, may suffer from many different dysrhythmias involving almost any rhythm or conduction disturbance [38–40]. The most common disorders are first-degree AV block or more advanced AV block degree and premature ventricular contractions.

Digoxin has two main actions in the cardiac myocyte: inhibition of the Na^+-K^+ Adenosinetryphosphate pump, interfering with AV conduction and increase in calcium concentrations, enhancing automaticity [41].

It is therefore important to recognize associated electrolyte disturbances, acid-base alterations, and renal or hepatic failure. In digoxin intoxication, hyperkalemia can be also sustained via a toxic mechanism of the Na^+-K^+ pump, which can be difficult to treat and can result after the treatment in hypokalemia.

In the presence of bradyarrhythmias, both atropine and cardiac pacing are usually effective. The most effective treatment for digitalis overdose is the administration of antidigitalis immunoglobulin IgG. The administration of magnesium and lidocaine often successfully treats premature ventricular contractions.

10.3.2.3 Antiarrhythmic Drugs

A patient with a history of atrial fibrillation treated with an antiarrhythmic drug such as flecainide or propafenone can present at the ED with an atrial flutter with a 2:1 or 1:1 atrioventricular conduction, or, in cases of drug abuse, also with a wide complex tachycardia related to class I effects on Na channels and QRS prolongation (Fig. 10.3).

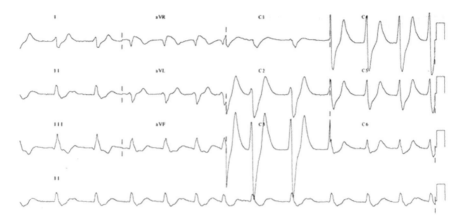

Fig. 10.3 A 60-year-old woman, 60 kg, with a history of paroxysmal atrial fibrillation; intake of 300 mg flecainide per os

10.3.2.4 Benzodiazepine

When a patient with a history of anxiety presents at the ED with palpitations, the medical history plays, as usual, an important role; in fact, discontinuation of benzo-diazepine (BDZ) can cause a withdrawal syndrome with reactions that vary in severity and duration. Withdrawal syndrome is more common with triazolam and BDZs with a short to intermediate half-life, in particular if taken in repeated doses during the day, whereas the syndrome is rare with long-half-life BDZs and virtually absent with BDZ analogues such as zolpidem and zopiclone.

Arrhythmias during withdrawal syndrome are induced by autonomic arousal caused by sympathetic hyperactivity, and include mainly sinus tachycardia and ectopic beats, often associated with blood pressure imbalance (orthostatic hypotension and mild systolic hypertension). The administration of β-blockers or clonidine can help in managing reactions resulting from sympathetic hyperactivity [42].

10.3.2.5 Antidepressant Agents

Depressed patients seem to be predisposed to cardiac arrhythmias, one of the proposed mechanisms involves a reduced parasympathetic nervous system activity, that can be often present as a decreased heart rate variability [43].

In patients with depression presenting with dysrhythmias in the ED, it is important to recognize the different classes of drugs.

- *Tricyclic antidepressant agents* (TCA), such as imipramine, amitriptyline, and clomipramine, act as nonselective monoamine reuptake inhibitors. TCAs induce quinidine-like effects that are frequently encountered in older patients and children. On surface ECG it's often recognizable an intraventricular block and atrio-ventricular conduction block of different degrees with an increase in QRS width and PR interval; moreover, there are repolarization abnormalities with QT interval prolongation and negative T waves: therefore these patients present with a higher risk of ventricular arrhythmias, in particular torsade de pointes. TCA can also induce sinus tachycardia (5–20 % of patients treated), with a mean increase of 15–20 bpm, probably caused by peripheral anticholinergic activity. Patients with cardiac diseases treated with class IC antiarrhythmic drugs (flecainide, propafenone) or quinidine should be closely monitored because the interaction between these drugs can lead to an increase in TCA blood concentration.

- *Selective serotonin reuptake inhibitors* (SSRI) include fluoxetine, sertraline, paroxetine, and citalopram, among others. A sinus tachycardia can be frequently recorded and, rarely, palpitations. In older patients SSRI can lead to sinus bradycardia and, rarely, syncope. In the case of drug overdose rhythm disorders, both bradyarrhythmia and tachyarrhythmia, as well as hypotension, are frequently present [44]. SSRI inhibits hepatic CYP3A4 and it is important to avoid or administer with reduced doses antiarrhythmic drugs as amiodarone, flecainide, propafenone, and lidocaine (i.v.) or sildenafil. [44, 45].

- *Monoamine oxidase inhibitors* (MAOI), such as phenelzine, tranylcypromine, and isocarboxazid, comprise the third main group of drugs used in clinical practice. A patient taking MAOI and presenting at the ED with palpitations and either tachycardia or bradycardia should be evaluated for a hypertensive surge, which has sometimes been reported as fatal. The anamnesis plays a pivotal role; in fact if the patient has ingested cheese or other foods with a high tyramine content, the arrhythmias could be due to norepinephrine release and an exaggerated adrenergic reaction induced by high tyramine blood levels [46–48].

10.3.2.6 Antibiotics

Patients treated with antibiotics can often present at the ED with sinus tachycardia or palpitations related to ectopic beats or to high rate atrial fibrillation; both dysrhythmias are probably related to the underlying condition (usually an infection) and subsequent fever and electrolyte disturbances.

In any event, a 12-lead ECG is mandatory to exclude a QTc prolongation and the risk of ventricular arrhythmias, in particular torsade de pointes.

These arrhythmias can be due to the following classes of antibiotics:

- *Macrolides* such as erythromycin, clarithromycin, and azithromycin. The risk of QT prolongation is higher if an H1 antagonist (e.g., terfenadine, astemizole) is administered at the same time. QT prolongation has been described with erythromycin, spiramycin and, less frequently, clarithromycin and azithromycin. Moreover, palpitations have been reported in patients taking azithromycin. An increase in digoxin levels has been reported in patients receiving erythromycin attributable to killing of digoxin-metabolizing bacteria [49].

- *Fluoroquinolones* such as levofloxacin and ciprofloxacin. Rarely, ventricular arrhythmias resulting from QT prolongation have been described during fluoroquinolone therapy.

10.4   A Suggested Algorithm/Pathway for Diagnosis and Treatment

All patients with bradyarrhythmia or tachyarrhythmia and suspected drug abuse or intoxication	What to do	How to do it
	Medical history and identification of suspected drug/s	Habitual medications Coexisting diseases Which substance or mix was taken (! alcohol) When the substance/mix was taken If a mix of substances was taken, which was the sequela Route of substance abuse: tablets, intravenous, inhalation, transdermal, sublingual
	Search for antidote	Contact local poison control center (the telephone number should be available in every ED)
	Medical management	Cardiopulmonary support including fluids DC shock if hemodynamically unstable arrhythmias or temporary pacing if bradycardia Gastrointestinal decontamination of an ingested drug Administration of an antidote if available Correction of acid–base and electrolyte alterations

References

1. Von Mach AA, Brinkmann X, Weilemann LS. Epidemiology of cardiac dysrhythmias in acute intoxication. Z Kardiol. 2004;93 Suppl 4:IV9–15.
2. European drug report 2014: trends and developments. http://www.emcdda.europa.eu.
3. Kesha K, Boggs CL, Ripple MG. Methylenedioxypyrovalerone (bath salts) related death: case report and review of the literature. J Forensic Sci. 2013;58(6):1654–9.
4. WADA list 2015, yearly updated www.wada-ama.org.
5. Tokish JM, Kocher MS, Hawkins RJ. Ergogenic aids: a review of basic science, performance, side effects, and status in sports. Am J Sports Med. 2004;32:1543–53.
6. Dhar R, Stout W, Link SM, Homoud MK, Weinstock J, Estes III M. Cardiovascular toxicities of performance-enhancing substances in sports. Mayo Clin Proc. 2005;80:1307–15.
7. Kutscher EC, Lund BC, Perry PJ. Anabolic steroids: a review for the clinician. Sports Med. 2002;32:285–96.
8. Gauthier J. The heart and doping. Arch Mal Coeur Vaiss. 2006;99:1126–9.

9. Calfee R, Fadale P. Popular ergogenic drugs and supplements in young athletes. Pediatrics. 2006;117:577–89.
10. Bouchard R, Weber AR, Geiger JD. Informed decision-making on sympathomimetic use in sport and health. Clin J Sport Med. 2002;12:209–24.
11. Gray SD, Fatovich DM, McCoubrie DL, Daly FF. Amphetamine-related presentations to an inner-city tertiary emergency department: a prospective evaluation. Med J Aust. 2007;186:336–9.
12. Krome CN, Tucker AM. Cardiac arrhythmia in a professional football player. Was ephedrine to blame? Phys Sports Med. 2003;31:1–12.
13. Gee P, Richardson S, Woltersdorf W, Moore G. Toxic effects of BZP-based herbal party pills in humans: a prospective study in Christchurch, New Zealand. NZ Med J. 2005;18:1227–37.
14. Hall AP, Henry JA. Acute toxic effects of "Ecstasy" (MDMA and related compounds: overview of pathophysiology and clinical management. Br J Anaesth. 2006;96:678–85.
15. Ricaurte GA, McCann UD. Recognition and management of complications of new recreational drug use. Lancet. 2005;365:2137–45.
16. Haller CA, Benowitz NL. Adverse cardiovascular and central nervous system events associated with dietary supplements containing ephedra alkaloids. N Engl J Med. 2000;343:1833–8.
17. Zahn KA, Li RL, Purssell RA. Cardiovascular toxicity after ingestion of 'herbal ecstasy'. J Emerg Med. 1999;17:289–91.
18. Furlanello F, Vitali Serdoz L, Cappato R, De Ambroggi L. Illicit drugs and cardiac arrhythmias in athletes. Eur J Cardiovasc Prev Rehabil. 2007;14:487–94.
19. Hunterdon Drug Awareness Program (HDAP). Comprehensive drug information on "bath salts" (MDPV, Mephedrone). Flemington: HDAP. Updated 29 June 2012; http://www.hdap.org/mdpv.html.
20. Benzie F, Hekman K, Cameron L, Wade DR, Miller C, Smolinske S, et al. Emergency department visits after use of a drug sold as "bath salts"–Michigan, November 13, 2010-March 31, 2011. MMWR Morb Mortal Wkly Rep. 2011;19:624–47.
21. Billman GE. Cocaine: a review of its toxic actions on cardiac function. Crit Rev Toxicol. 1995;25:113–32.
22. Karch SB. Cocaine cardiovascular toxicity. South Med J. 2005;98:794–9.
23. Kloner RA, Hale S, Alker K, Rezkalla S. The effects of acute and chronic cocaine use on the heart. Circulation. 1992;85:407–19.
24. Hale SL, Lehmann MH, Kloner RA. Electrocardiographic abnormalities after acute administration of cocaine in the rat. Am J Cardiol. 1989;63:1529–30.
25. Taylor D, Paroish D, Thompson K, Cavaliere M. Cocaine induced prolongation of the QT interval. Emerg Med J. 2004;21:252–3.
26. Magnano AR, Talathoti NB, Hallur R, Jurus DT, Dizon J, Holleran S, et al. Effect of Acute Cocaine Administration on the QTc Interval of Habitual Users. Am J Cardiol. 2006;97:1244–6.
27. Fuller TE, Milling TJ, Price B, Spangle K. Therapeutic hypothermia in cocaine-induced cardiac arrest. Ann Emerg Med. 2008;51:135–7.
28. Hollander JE, Hoffman RS. Cocaine-induced myocardial infarction: an analysis and review of the literature. J Emerg Med. 1992;10:169–77.
29. Turhan H, Aksoy Y, Ozgun Tekin G, Yetkin E. Cocaine-induced acute myocardial infarction in young individuals with otherwise normal coronary risk profile: is coronary microvascular dysfunction one of the underlying mechanisms? Int J Cardiol. 2007;114:106–7.
30. Mittleman MA, Mintzer D, Maclure M, Togler GH, Sherwood JB, Muller JE. Triggering of myocardial infarction by cocaine. Circulation. 1999;99:2737–41.
31. Guo J, Gang H, Zhang S. Molecular determinants of cocaine block of human ether-a-go-go-related gene potassium channels. J Pharmacol Exp Ther. 2006;317:865–74.
32. Parker RB, Perry GY, Horan LG, Flowers NC. Comparative effects of sodium bicarbonate and sodium chloride on reversing cocaine-induced changes in the electrocardiogram. J Cardiovasc Pharmacol. 1999;34:864–9.

33. Littmann L, Monroe MH, Svenson RH. Brugada-type electrocardiographic pattern induced by cocaine. Mayo Clin Proc. 2000;75:845–9.
34. Randall T. Cocaine, alcohol mix in body to form even longer lasting, more lethal drug. JAMA. 1992;267:1043–4.
35. Lindsay AC, Foale RA, Warren O, Henry JA. Cannabis as a precipitant of cardiovascular emergencies. Int J Cardiol. 2005;104:230–2.
36. Fisher BA, Ghuran A, Vadamalai V, Antonios TF. Cardiovascular complications induced by cannabis smoking: a case report and review of the literature. Emerg Med J. 2005;22:679–80.
37. Aryana A, Williams MA. Marijuana as a trigger of cardiovascular events: speculation or scientific certainty? Int J Cardiol. 2007;118:141–4.
38. Pita-Fernandez S, Lombardia-Cortina M, Orozco-Veltran D, Gil-Guillen V. Clinical manifestations of elderly patients with digitalis intoxication in the emergency department. Arch Geron Geriat. 2011;53:e106–10.
39. Davis JA, Ravishanktar C, Shah MJ. Multiple cardiac arrhythmias in a previously healthy child: a case of accidental digitalis intoxication. Pediatr Emerg Care. 2006;22(6):430–4.
40. Goranitou G, Stavrianaki D, Babalis D. Wide QRS tachycardia caused by severe hyperkalaemia and digoxin intoxication. Acta Cardiol. 2005;60(4):437–41.
41. Deret RW, Horowitz BZ. Cardiotoxic drugs. Emerg Med Clin North Am. 1995;13:771–91.
42. Shader RI, Greenblatt DJ. Use of benzodiazepines in anxiety disorders. N Engl J Med. 1993;328(19):1398–405.
43. Mann JJ. The medical management of depression. N Engl J Med. 2005;353(17):1819–34.
44. Shader RI, Greenblatt DJ. Selective serotonin reuptake inhibitor antidepressants: cardiovascular complications-sorting through findings. J Clin Psychopharmacol. 2001;21(5):467–8.
45. Warrington SJ, Padgham C, Lader M. The cardiovascular effects of antidepressants. Psychol Med Monogr Suppl. 1989;16:i–iii, 1–40.
46. Yamada M, Yasuhara H. Clinical pharmacology of MAO inhibitors: safety and future. Neurotoxicology. 2004;25(1–2):215–21. Review.
47. Goldman LS, Alexander RC, Luchins DJ. Monoamine oxidase inhibitors and tricyclic antidepressants: comparison of their cardiovascular effects. J Clin Psychiatry. 1986;47(5):225–9.
48. Murray JB. Cardiac disorders and antidepressant medications. J Psychol. 2000;134(2):162–8. Review.
49. Periti P, Mazzei T, Mini E, Novelli A. Adverse effects of macrolide antibacterials. Drug Saf. 1993;9(5):346–64.

Pacemaker Malfunction: Myth or Reality?

11

Roberto Verlato, Maria Stella Baccillieri, and Pietro Turrini

11.1 Focusing on the Issue

Pacemaker (PM) and implantable cardiac defibrillator (ICD) malfunction is a serious and frequent finding in clinical setting. Depending on baseline rhythm and the type of malfunction, symptoms with different severity can occur, from no symptoms to syncope and sudden death due to asystole or ventricular fibrillation. Unfortunately, symptoms, such as asthenia, dizziness, dyspnea, and palpitations, are often vague, and this can lead to a dangerous delay in cardiac implantable electronic device (CIED) malfunction detection. An ECG recording and careful device and lead evaluation by means of telemetry are necessary for the diagnosis. A great help to early detection of CIED malfunctions is coming from remote control, allowing therapeutic interventions within 24 h since the malfunction occurs in most cases.

CIED malfunctions include two main categories: problems with sensing and problems with pacing. Problems with sensing are made of failure to sense, or *undersensing*, and excessive sensing of noncardiac or cardiac signals, called *oversensing*. Undersensing causes asynchronous inappropriate and not necessary pacing, which in turn can precipitate ventricular arrhythmias due to pacing during the ventricular refractory period (R-on-T phenomenon). Oversensing of spurious signals will lead to lack of stimulation and asystole in PM-dependent patients. In ICDs, inappropriate shocks are frequently caused by oversensing. Undersensing and oversensing are mostly due to lead-related problems, either insulation failure or conductor fractures. A connection defect must be considered as differential diagnosis. The problems with pacing have a common final result: PM spikes ineffective to capture the myocardium. If such malfunction is of minor importance in the atrium, it is a life-threatening emergency in PM-dependent patients, which can exit in sudden death.

R. Verlato, MD (✉) • M.S. Baccillieri, MD • P. Turrini, MD
Cardiology Unit, Hospital P. Cosma, Camposampiero, Padova, Italy
e-mail: roberto.verlato@libero.it

© Springer International Publishing Switzerland 2016
M. Zecchin, G. Sinagra (eds.), *The Arrhythmic Patient in the Emergency
Department: A Practical Guide for Cardiologists and Emergency Physicians*,
DOI 10.1007/978-3-319-24328-3_11

In patients with an implanted biventricular PM or ICD for cardiac resynchronization therapy (CRT), the loss of left ventricular capture is associated with recurrence of heart failure symptoms.

Battery depletion can lead to asynchronous pacing and other functional abnormalities mimicking either under- and oversensing.

11.2 What Physicians Working in Emergency Department Should Know

11.2.1 About Basic Function of Pacemakers and ECG Interpretation

The basics of PM are illustrated in Fig. 11.1, showing the normal function of a dual chamber (DDD) PM. These systems are preferred by cardiologists as they reproduce the normal atrioventricular (AV) conduction and physiology. They can sense and pace both the atrium and the ventricle. When they sense an atrial signal, a ventricular impulse is delivered at the end of the programmed AV delay. If no atrial signal is detected at the end of the programmed escape interval, the atrium is paced. If a ventricular spontaneous signal is sensed within the AV delay, no ventricular impulse is delivered to the ventricle [1].

The basics of single chamber (SSI), more often ventricular (VVI) PM, are more simple: the ventricle is paced at the end of the programmed escape interval, or basic rate, when nonsensed signal occurs within this time. In rate-responsive PM, either VVI or DDD, the stimulation rate is increased during effort according with sensors [1].

11.2.2 Most Important, Basic Programmable Functions in a Pacemaker

(a) *Lower rate*: it is the rate below which the pacemaker will stimulate the heart. If spontaneous activity is higher than the programmed lower rate, pacemaker output is inhibited. If programmed rate is higher than spontaneous rate and PM spikes are not visible, a malfunction is present, usually oversensing. The only exception is the presence of a "hysteresis" algorithm programmed on.

(b) *Hysteresis*: if this function is activated, the lower heart rate below which the PM will start the stimulation is different from the programmed pacing lower rate. For example, if hysteresis is programmed at 40/min and lower rate at 70/min, the PM will start the stimulation only if spontaneous heart rate drops below 40/min, but stimulation rate will be 70/min. The PM will check periodically the presence of spontaneous rate between 40 and 70/min.

(c) *Rate-responsive pacing*: the stimulation rate is increased when activity sensors detect patient movements (accelerometers). Respiratory activity sensors or other algorithms are also able to increase the basic pacing rate.

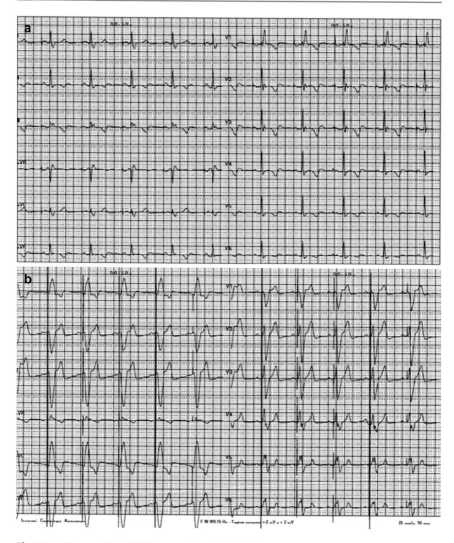

Fig. 11.1 *Top panel* (**a**). DDD pacemaker. Atrial rhythm is paced at 60 bpm. Spontaneous QRS with right bundle branch morphology occurs after 180 ms that inhibits ventricular pacing. This is called atrial-driven rhythm. *Bottom panel* (**b**): spontaneous sinus rhythm is present; each P wave is followed by a ventricular stimulus at the end of the programmed AV delay (120 ms) that captures the ventricular myocardium. The QRS morphology is left bundle branch block with superior axis, typical of right ventricular apical pacing

(d) *Upper rate*: it is the maximum stimulation rate either in case of atrial-driven or sensor-driven stimulation. If the PM stimulates at a rate higher than the programmed upper rate, a hardware/software malfunction is present. This can happen in case of unprotected exposition to strong electromagnetic fields, such as magnetic resonance imaging.

(e) *Algorithms to reduce ventricular pacing:* in order to reduce unnecessary ventricular pacing, several algorithms are present in modern dual chamber PM. Most commonly, only the atrium is stimulated (AAI mode) if atrioventricular conduction is preserved; when one or two (depending on the model and device programming) consecutive A-V blocks occur, the mode of stimulation automatically changes to atrioventricular pacing (DDD mode). Other algorithms prolong the programmed A-V interval up to 400 ms to detect if spontaneous A-V conduction is present. When these algorithms are activated, it is sometimes difficult to understand if the PM is working normally or not, for example, in case of single atrial beats without any ventricular activity; this can be a normal behavior of the device, when followed by DDD pacing, but can be expression of ventricular oversensing. Knowledge of the device programming, PM interrogation, or real-time telemetry can be necessary for the diagnosis.

(f) *Pacing voltage*: this is the voltage of PM stimulus. If it is programmed below the ventricular pacing threshold, spikes will be ineffective leading to an *exit block*.

(g) *Pulse duration*: this is the duration of PM stimulus. If it is programmed too short, spikes could be ineffective leading to an exit block.

(h) *Autocapture*: this algorithms automatically reduce PM output energy to values just above the ventricular pacing threshold. In case the delivered stimulus doesn't capture the ventricle, a second high-energy stimulus is provided: this is a normal behavior of modern PM and not a malfunction.

(i) *Mode switch*: when this algorithms are activated in dual chamber PM, the mode of stimulation automatically switches from DDD(R) to VDI(R) when an atrial tachycardia/fibrillation is detected. If atrial arrhythmia terminates, the mode of stimulation will return from VDI to DDD [1].

11.3   What Cardiologists Should Know

Cardiologists must be familiar with basic PM functions, mode of stimulation, PM algorithms, and interpretation of ECG recordings in PM patients. Modern PMs are very complex, fully programmable devices, with a lot of therapeutic and diagnostic capabilities. PM interrogation, evaluation of battery and lead data, analysis of real-time telemetry, and stored data are necessary for the final evaluation of PM functions. It would be desirable that cardiologists were trained and capable to use at least basic functions of PM programmers and the meaning and utilization of the following:

(a) *Magnet*: the application of a magnet above the PM pocket induces asynchronous pacing (VOO or DOO in single chamber or dual chamber PM, respectively). In case a PM is apparently not working (because spikes are not evident) but bradycardia (below lower rate, including hysteresis) is present, it is useful to apply a magnet on the PM. If PM spikes appear and capture the ventricle, oversensing inhibiting PM stimulation is likely. When necessary, in this cases magnet function is also useful for emergency treatment of the bradycardia.

(b) *ERI*: this is a message of "low battery charge" (Elective Replacement Indicator), meaning that the device will soon (usually after about 3 months) reaches the complete battery depletion, or EOL (End Of Life); ERT (Elective Replacement Time) and EOS (End Of Service) are synonymous of ERI and EOL, respectively, used by some manufacturers.

(c) *Pacing impedance*: this value is normally in the range between 350 and 900 Ω. Pacing impedance is influenced by the integrity of pacing circuit (conductors and insulation), by the lead model (i.e., active or passive fixation, steroid eluting or normal electrodes), and by electrode endocardial contact surface. When pacing impedance drops below 250 Ω, an insulation failure of the lead is likely. When pacing impedance is above 1500–2000 Ω (depending on the lead model), a conductor fracture or a connection defect is possibly present. In case of an abnormal pacing impedance in bipolar pacing and sensing configuration, PM reprogramming to unipolar pacing and sensing is recommended.

All cardiologists involved in emergency evaluation of PM patients should be trained to recognize the most commonly PM malfunctions, i.e., undersensing, oversensing, and exit block [1–3].

11.3.1 Undersensing in Cardiac Pacemakers

Undersensing occurs when the PM fails to sense the spontaneous atrial or ventricular activity. In this case the PM will ignore the spontaneous activity and pace the heart at the programmed rate as if the patient had no rhythm. This results in the so-called "asynchronous" pacing, that is, pacing competitive with spontaneous cardiac activity. Ventricular pacing during the vulnerable period of cardiac cycle (T wave) can occur, triggering ventricular arrhythmias including ventricular fibrillation [1–3].

An example of ventricular undersensing is illustrated in Fig. 11.2.

11.3.1.1 Causes of Undersensing

Causes of undersensing include lead failure, pacemaker failure, and environmental and physiologic changes. Lead failure is the most frequent cause of under- and oversensing in current CIEDs. Both insulation failure and lead fracture are able to induce undersensing, so it is pivotal to interrogate the pacemaker to evaluate pacing impedance. An increase of pacing impedance > 2000 Ω is diagnostic of conductor damage. A decrease of pacing impedance below 250 Ω is diagnostic of insulation failure. A connection defect is usually associated with a high pacing impedance, >3000 Ω, and this must be distinguished from conduction fracture in the presence of high pacing impedances. To identify a connection defect, chest X-ray is useful, as it can show the lead connector incompletely inserted into the PM head. An example of connection defect is illustrated in Fig. 11.3.

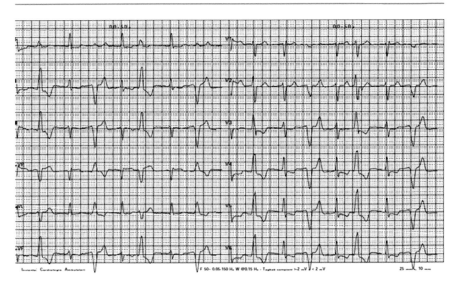

Fig. 11.2 VVI pacemaker. Spontaneous rhythm is present interrupted by premature beats of different morphology. At careful ECG inspection, small pacemaker spikes (bipolar) precede the QRS with left bundle branch morphology and left axis deviation. Other spikes follow spontaneous QRS in random sequence (asynchronous pacing). Undersensing of ventricular activity is present

Fig. 11.3 Chest X-ray showing a close-up of pacemaker pocket. Patient had undergone to device replacement 1 week before and presented with high pacing impedance (>3000 Ω), under- and oversensing. The connector of the atrial lead, the lateral one, is completely inserted into the head of pacemaker, and its terminal pin is visible outside the electrode ring. The ventricular connector (*arrow*) is incompletely inserted and its terminal end is not visible

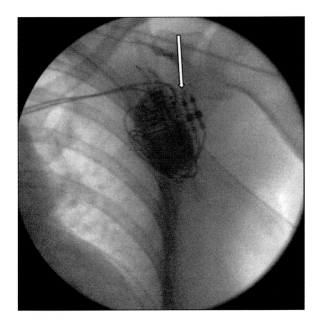

Chest X-ray is less useful to detect lead failure as leads seem apparently intact in most cases.

Pacemaker failure can cause undersensing. The most frequent situation is battery depletion (end of service, or EOL message at telemetry interrogation is displayed): this switches the mode of stimulation to asynchronous pacing.

Environmental causes of undersensing are strong magnetic fields, such as anti-theft devices, great motor engines, the application of a magnet on the pacemaker pocket, and magnetic resonance imaging. A frequent environment cause of undersensing is cardiac defibrillation. In this case undersensing but also an exit block with lack of ventricular capture can occur due to tissue damage at the myocardium-tip electrode interface.

Physiologic cardiac and noncardiac changes can facilitate undersensing, reducing the amplitude of cardiac sensed signals. New bundle branch block, myocardial infarction, hypokalemia and other ionic abnormalities, and old age of the implanted lead, associated with fibrous tissue growing around the electrode tip, are all situations associated with PM undersensing.

11.3.1.2 Treatment of PM Undersensing

In the case of reduced amplitude of sensed signals (measured by telemetry), it's possible to increase the PM sensing function by reprogramming, even if this in turn increases the risk of oversensing, in particular for unipolar leads. PM or lead replacement is the only way to correct the malfunction when battery depletion or lead failure is present [1–3].

11.3.2 Undersensing in ICDs

Undersensing in ICDs recognizes the same causes as in cardiac PM. Lead failure, either insulation or conductor defects, is the most dangerous situation in ICD patients, and it must be excluded in the presence of undersensing or oversensing. In ICDs either lead-related undersensing or oversensing may be intermittent, making diagnosis more difficult. A "physiologic" degree of undersensing is frequently observed in ICDs due to low voltages of cardiac signals during ventricular tachycardia and fibrillation, but this is rarely a clinical problem. Otherwise, prolonged ventricular undersensing during ventricular fibrillation (VF) could result in patient death, and the only possible treatment is an external rescue shock. However, in ICDs the most frequent cause of ventricular tachycardia (VT) undersensing is a programming "error," that is, the cutoff detection rate set at values above the rate of spontaneous VT. Reprogramming of VT detection rate will correct the problem [1].

11.3.3 Oversensing in Cardiac Pacemakers

Oversensing occurs when a PM senses noise, artifacts, or physiologic cardiac or noncardiac signals different from the atrial or ventricular depolarization and classifies such signals as atrial or ventricular depolarizations. The result will be inhibition of ventricular pacing when oversensing occurs at ventricular level or unnecessary ventricular pacing when oversensing occurs at atrial level. Pacing during oversensing is erratic, irregular, and completely unrelated with the programmed lower rate. In the case of prolonged pacing inhibition in PM-dependent patients, asystole will occur [1–3].

11.3.3.1 Causes of Oversensing

Lead failure is by far the most frequent cause of oversensing. Insulation failure, conductor fracture, and lead dislodgement are all able to induce oversensing of noise. Lead problems are identified by means of pacing impedance measurements, as described for undersensing. High pacing impedance is diagnostic of conductor problems, low impedance of insulation defect. Lead dislodgement and connection defect are often visible on X-ray imaging.

Environmental electromagnetic interferences (EMI) are the second more frequent cause of oversensing. They can reach the distal dipole of PM leads because electromagnetic currents flow through the patient's body, which acts as a volume conductor. Electrocautery, extracorporeal shock lithotripsy, and MRI (when CIED presence is ignored) are frequent causes of oversensing in the hospital setting. Noise signals can also originate from metal to metal friction in patients with multiple implanted pacemaker or defibrillation leads.

Myopotential oversensing can occur at pocket level (pectoral muscle oversensing), especially when programmed unipolar sensing, but more frequently the PM can sense the diaphragmatic respiratory activity.

T wave oversensing is the most common situation of oversensing of cardiac physiologic signals; it leads to a decrease of pacing rate as the escape interval is reset by the T wave sensing [1–3].

11.3.3.2 Treatment of Oversensing

The application of a magnet on the pocket will immediately induce (in PM, not in ICDs) atrial and ventricular asynchronous pacing. In the emergency setting this is the only maneuver that must be immediately applied to the patient, especially if symptomatic bradycardia is present.

If the PM programmer is available, sensing function must be reprogrammed to decrease PM sensitivity. In the case of unipolar sensing, the change of sensing configuration to bipolar, if a bipolar lead is implanted, will reduce or even could completely correct the oversensing of muscle potentials. In case T wave oversensing is present, longer ventricular refractory periods must be programmed.

The switch of pacing mode to VOO, or asynchronous, is the safest option in PM-dependent patients with oversensing due to lead problems to correct the bradycardia. In this case replacement of the failing lead is mandatory [1–3].

11.3.4 Oversensing in ICDs

Oversensing is the second leading cause of inappropriate detection and therapy of arrhythmias, including inappropriate shocks after atrial tachyarrhythmias. Lead failure must be suspected in any case of inappropriate shocks and noise stored in device memories. Several algorithms have been developed for early detection of lead failure based on the presence of very short intervals between sensed signals. The presence of a connection defect must always be considered as an alternative source of noise oversensing. Failing ICD leads must be replaced, with or without lead extraction based on careful evaluation of individual risk/benefit profile of lead extraction.

When noise oversensing is due to interference between implanted leads, lead extraction is mandatory [1–4].

11.3.5 Problems with Pacing

The most frequent situation is the presence of pacemaker spikes visible on monitor screens or ECG recordings, not followed by ventricular or atrial depolarizations (exit block). The failure to capture must be immediately recognized as it is a life-threatening malfunction.

In Fig. 11.4 an example of failure to capture is shown. PM spikes are delivered by pulse generator, not followed by ventricular depolarization [1–3].

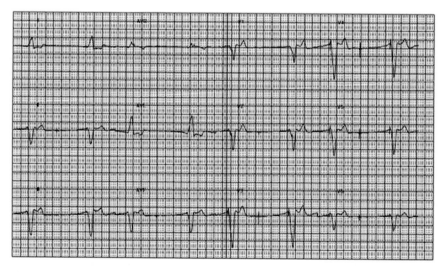

Fig. 11.4 Patient with PM presenting to the emergency room after a syncope. 12-lead ECG shows several pacemaker spikes not followed by ventricular depolarization (exit block). A failure to capture is certainly present. Real-time telemetry showed high pacing impedance (2500 Ω). Combining the two findings of exit block plus high pacing impedance, the diagnosis of lead fracture was made. Lead replacement was necessary in this case

11.3.5.1 Causes of Failure to Capture

In the period just following pacemaker implantation, lead dislodgement and cardiac perforation are the most common causes of failure to capture. Chest X-ray is necessary for the diagnosis, and reintervention for lead repositioning must be performed as soon as possible. Sometimes perforation is subtle, and a CT scan can be helpful to identify the relationship and exact position of the electrocatheter tip and the pericardium.

If the exit block occurs several weeks after implantation (the most frequent situation), it is usually due to an increase in stimulation threshold because of fibrosis maturation close and around to the electrode tip. Steroid-eluting leads are less frequently involved, while the risk is higher for active fixation leads, where an increase of pacing threshold frequently occurs during the first weeks after implantation. Such increase is usually transient, although it can rarely persist or even worsen (especially in young people) during follow-up.

Failure to capture can be also caused by too low voltage and/or duration of the stimulus emitted by the pacemaker in proximity of battery end of life or in the case of battery failure, but usually it depends by an inappropriate PM programming. Autocapture algorithms in modern pacemaker ensure ventricular capture.

Cardiac defibrillation and strong electromagnetic fields emitted by MRI can cause exit block due to tissue damage by current flow through the lead up to the electrodes, a sort of inadvertent tissue ablation, in particular when insulation failure is present.

Lead failure, in PM and especially in ICDs, is very often associated with deterioration of pacing and sensing thresholds, in addition with under- and oversensing [1–3].

11.3.5.2 Treatment of Failure to Capture

Acute perforation usually presents as an emergency in operating room. It requires pericardiocentesis and immediate lead repositioning.

Subacute and chronic perforation may be difficult to recognize. Symptoms may be minor; pericarditis, chest pain, diaphragmatic stimulation, and sometimes pneumothorax may be present. Perforation may occur at both atrial and ventricular levels. Loss of capture is almost always present together with sensing problems. Device reprogramming can transiently be useful to correct sensing and pacing abnormalities, but again lead revision/repositioning is absolutely required to solve the problem once the diagnosis is made.

When failure to capture occurs due to increased pacing thresholds, device reprogramming and selection of higher energy output, in terms of pulse voltage and duration, are the solutions in the acute setting. However, in current pacemaker technologies, the programmation of high pacing energies, i.e., voltage amplitude of 5–6 V and pulse duration of 1–2 ms, is associated with a marked reduction of battery longevity, up to less than two years. Lead revision, reposition, or replacement must be considered in pacemaker-dependent and/or young people with high pacing threshold.

Failure to capture occurring after MRI or cardiac defibrillation requires lead revision.

11.4   False Malfunctions

In modern devices, the complexity of some algorithms can sometimes make the ECG interpretation and the distinction between normal behavior and malfunctions quite difficult.

For this reason, to reach a correct ECG interpretation, it is necessary to know the model and the programming of the device, because what can be considered a normal behavior in some models and with some programming can be a malfunction in other cases [5].

- For example, a spontaneous rate below the lower rate programmed can be normal when a hysteresis is programmed, but a marker of oversensing in the absence of this function.
- In order to prevent sudden changes of the heart rate, an algorithm called "rate smoothing", "flywheel" or "ventricular rate stabilization," according to the man- ufacturer, can be enabled. In this case, stimulation can transiently occur beyond the lower rate, even if a rate response function is not present, just after a sponta- neous fast activity, allowing a "smooth" reduction of heart rate. This can fre- quently happen during atrial fibrillation with very irregular rate, after ectopic ventricular beats or at the end of a tachycardia.
- Convincing data have shown that stimulation of the right ventricle is hemody- namically unfavorable and can sometimes cause or worsen congestive heart fail- ure. In some devices, algorithms for minimizing ventricular pacing are enabled. In this case it is possible to observe an extremely long PQ interval, or even two consecutive P waves (spontaneous or stimulated) not followed by any ventricular activity, before the automatic switch from AAI (or ADI) to DDD mode occurs (Fig. 11.5).

Finally, a very short paced AV interval (about 100 ms) can sometimes be observed.

This is due to a function called "ventricular safety pacing," which consists in the delivery of a ventricular stimulus when a signal is detected in the ventricular channel immediately after an atrial stimulation. As in practice, the device is not able to distinguish whether the signal is derived by the artifact of atrial pacing detected at ventricular level (crosstalk) or a real ventricular beat (as an ectopic ventricular beat), so it immediately delivers a ventricular stimulus ensuring stimu- lation (in the presence of crosstalk) but with an interval short enough to fall, in the presence of a beat of ventricular origin, in its refractory period, avoiding the risk of triggering dangerous arrhythmias. Ventricular safety pacing can be present even in case of a lack of atrial sensing, when the atrial stimulus coincides with the spontaneous QRS complex, as in the course of sinus rhythm and normal AV conduction.

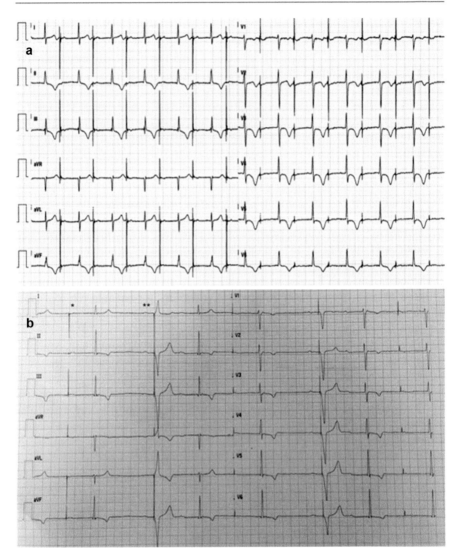

Fig. 11.5 Apparent malfunctions due to algorithm for reduction of ventricular pacing. (**a**) Atrial stimulation with spontaneous AV conduction with very long (440 ms) PQ interval. (**b**) Alternation of AAI (*) and DDD (**) mode, resulting in excessively low ventricular rate

11.5 What to Do in Case a Pacemaker Malfunction Is Suspected

If a PM malfunction is suspected, the patient must be immediately monitored and a complete standard 12-lead ECG obtained.

If artifacts of stimulation are not visible on ECG recording, a magnet must be applied on the device pocket. This will induce asynchronous pacing in both the atrium and ventricle (VOO, DOO). If pacemaker stimuli become visible, it will be possible to evaluate if they capture the heart (paced P waves and QRS).

If the bradycardia is corrected by magnet application, oversensing is present and lead failure must be considered the most likely cause. The main differential diagnosis is with the presence of a connection defect, especially if the patient has recently undergone PM replacement.

If PM artifacts are visible but fail to capture, either constantly or intermittently even with magnet application, lead dislodgment, cardiac perforation, lead failure, high pacing thresholds, tissue ablation, and programmation errors are the possible causes of the exit block.

Device control by means of real-time telemetry is essential for the final diagnosis. Pacing impedance instant value and trends must be examined. High or low pacing impedances (>2000 or <250 Ω) are diagnostics of lead failure. As they can be intermittent, the temporal impedance trends must be obtained as well. The presence of even only one out-of-range value allows the diagnosis of lead failure. Pacing and sensing thresholds may be evaluated in real time and temporal trends examined.

Battery level is immediately displayed on programmer screen after interrogation, and a message of alert is displayed if battery level is low (ERI, EOS, EOL messages).

Chest X-ray must be obtained to check for connection defects or visible lead fracture, in particular in ICDs recipients. If cardiac perforation is suspected, an echocardiogram and CT scan are recommended.

If a malfunction of the generator is present, like battery exhaustion, PM replacement is necessary. Lead revision/replacement reposition is necessary in most of the other cases as discussed above.

References

1. Ellenbogen KA, Kaszala K. Cardiac pacing and ICDs. 6th ed. Boston: Wiley-Blackwell Editors; 2014.
2. Harper RJ, Brady WJ, Perron AD, et al. The paced electrocardiogram: issues for emergency physicians. Am J Emerg Med. 2001;19:551–60.
3. Sarko JA, Tiffany BR. Cardiac Pacemakers: evaluation and management of malfunctions. Am J Emerg Med. 2004;18:435–40.
4. Wilkoff BL, Love CJ, Byrd CL, et al. Transvenous lead extraction: HRS expert consensus on facilities, training, indications and patient management. Heart Rhythm. 2009;6:1085–104.
5. Lloyd MS, El Chami NF, Langberg JJ. Pacing features that mimic malfunction: a review of current programmable and automated device functions that cause confusion in the clinical setting. J Cardiovasc Electrophysiol. 2009;20:453–60.

Management of the Electrical Storm in Patients with ICD

12

Daniele Muser, Domenico Facchin, Luca Rebellato, and Alessandro Proclemer

12.1 Focusing on the Issue

Current definition of electrical storm (ES) is the occurrence of three or more episodes of sustained ventricular tachycardia (VT) or ventricular fibrillation (VF) within 24 h requiring appropriate medical intervention. The same definition applies in implantable cardioverter-defibrillator (ICD) carriers in which ES is defined by three or more appropriate and separate (at least 5 min) device interventions in 24 h, either with antitachycardia pacing (ATP) or shock [1].

Current guidelines recommend ICD implantation for secondary prevention of sudden cardiac death (SCD) in survivors of cardiac arrest with no correctable causes and in patients with sustained symptomatic VT of different etiology. They also recommend ICD implantation for primary prevention in patients with ischemic or non-ischemic dilated cardiomyopathy and ejection fraction equal or lower than 35 % after at least 3 months of optimized medical therapy [2] and in other less frequent inherited arrhythmogenic syndromes.

Considering that approximately 1–2 % of the adult population in developed countries suffer from heart failure (HF) and that at least half of these patients have a low ejection fraction [3], the number of ICD carriers is wide spreading. Moreover, the improving therapies of HF ensure a long survival of patients making them older and affected by more comorbidities. For these reasons, ES is an increasingly

D. Muser
Clinical Cardiac Electrophysiology, Hospital of the University of Pennsylvania, Philadelphia, PA, USA

D. Facchin • L. Rebellato • A. Proclemer (✉)
Cardiology Unit, Santa Maria Della Misericordia University Hospital, Udine, Italy
e-mail: proclemer.alessandro@aoud.sanita.fvg.it

© Springer International Publishing Switzerland 2016
M. Zecchin, G. Sinagra (eds.), *The Arrhythmic Patient in the Emergency Department: A Practical Guide for Cardiologists and Emergency Physicians*, DOI 10.1007/978-3-319-24328-3_12

frequent cause of access to emergency department (ED). It is estimated that about 25 % of ICD carriers experience at least one ES episode per year follow-up [4]. ES is definitely a medical emergency requiring a multidisciplinary approach.

12.2 What Physicians Working in ED and Anesthesiologists Should Know

12.2.1 How Is an ICD Made and How Does It Work?

The ICD is a subcutaneous implantable device able to monitor cardiac rhythm and terminate potentially life-threatening arrhythmias. It consists of two main components:

- The *generator* that contains the battery, all the circuits that run the device, and the operator communicating system. It is implanted in a subcutaneous pocket, usually under the left clavicle.
- The *leads* that reach heart chambers through the venous system and allow the device to either monitor heart electrical activity and deliver therapies. The ICDs have a lead implanted in the right ventricle apex able both to record ventricular activity and release therapies like pacing and/or direct current shock. In adjunct some ICDs have another lead implanted in the right atrium to record atrial electrical activity, improving discrimination between supraventricular arrhythmias (SVA) and ventricular ones and to pace the atrium (ICD-DR). ICDs with cardiac resynchronization therapy (CRT-D) have a third lead that paces the left ventricle, through the coronary venous system, synchronously to the right ventricle improving contractility. Some recent devices are implanted entirely subcutaneously, leads included (subcutaneous ICD), and can deliver high-energy shocks only (without long-term pacing capabilities) without a direct contact with the heart chambers and no leads inserted in the venous system.

ICDs use mathematical algorithms defined by the manufacturer to discriminate life-threatening ventricular arrhythmias from SVA and deliver appropriate therapy. Sometimes correct recognition fails, and in this case the therapy delivered is defined *inappropriate*. In other cases the delivered therapy may not be able to terminate the ventricular arrhythmia, and in this case it is called *ineffective*:

- The operator interfaces with the ICD through a programmer able to communicate with the device. Each manufacturer uses a different programmer, so it is imperative *to know the manufacturer and use the right equipment*. The programmer establishes an initial connection with the device through a head which must be positioned on the skin above the ICD. Usually green lights turn on to indicate the head is in the right place. At this point, depending on the features of the device, it may be necessary to maintain the head above the ICD throughout the query to allow communication, or, in some devices, the head can be removed since the communication continues via Wi-Fi.

The programmer allows the operator to visualize all the data stored in the device such as:

- *Arrhythmic events*: the device registers all arrhythmic events recognized as such on the basis of user-defined criteria. Each event provides endocavitary (or external for subcutaneous ICDs) electrocardiogram lead recording and therapies delivered.
- *Battery status.*
- Information about *lead integrity*.

On the basis of stored data, the operator may decide to change some settings such as:

- Arrhythmia recognition criteria (heart rate, time before treatment, algorithms for SVT recognition, etc.) and intervention criteria
- Type and characteristics of therapies delivered

12.2.2 How Does the ICD Recognize and Treat Arrhythmias (Appropriate Therapies)?

VT recognition is primarily based upon tachycardia cycle length (to distinguish from normal sinus rhythm) and duration (to detect non-sustained episodes). Both of these parameters are tailored on the patient's characteristics. Thus, ICD uses ventricular rate zones for rhythm classification. The boundaries between zones are defined by two main principles:

- The recognition of unstable fast VT/VF must be highly sensitive even at the cost of inappropriate rapid SVA treatment.
- The recognition of slower VT (generally better tolerated) has to be more specific to avoid inappropriate therapies even at the cost of some delay in detection.

The ICDs treat ventricular tachyarrhythmias by:

- *Antitachycardia pacing (ATP)*: it is a brief ventricular pacing (6–8 beats) with a cycle length slightly lower (thus at a faster rate) of the arrhythmia (usually 81–88 %), in the attempt of resetting the reentrant circuit and interrupting the arrhythmia. Sometimes the paced cycle shortens from beat to beat, and in this case it is referred as ATP ramp.
- *Direct current shock (DC shock)*: it is a biphasic electrical shock provided between the generator case and the coil localized on the right ventricular lead. The energy released may vary, reaching up to 40 J with the latest generation high-energy devices.

Basing on several studies [5–7], ICD programming should empirically involve the use of three rate zones:

- A slow VT zone up to 320 ms cycle length (<188 bpm)
- A fast VT zone from 320 to 240 ms (188–250 bpm)
- A VF zone from 240 ms (>250 bpm)

In both VT zones, a variable number of ATP attempts precede shocks delivery. In the slow VT zone, a greater number than in fast VT zone are usually programmed (e.g., 3 ATPs followed by 3 ATP ramps), as fast arrhythmias are usually less tolerated.

In the VF zone, the hemodynamic instability of the arrhythmia and its high life-threatening potential require an immediate shock delivery (usually at the maximum energy from the beginning). In modern devices an ATP during capacitor charging (usually requiring less than 10 s) is delivered, avoiding the shock in the case of arrhythmic interruption.

VT/VF detection not only is based upon ventricular rate but also requires a programmable duration of the arrhythmia to avoid detection of non-sustained episodes. Usually a VT/VF is detected when a certain percentage of ventricular sensed beats meets cycle length criteria. The type of counting used varies between detection zones and among manufacturers. In order to improve sensibility, according to some manufacturers, the arrhythmia is detected when a certain percentage of beats (not necessarily consecutive) falls in VF zone, while consecutive interval counting is required in the VT zone, increasing specificity. The time to detection in the VT zone should be longer enough to allow spontaneous termination of non-sustained episodes [6, 8].

12.2.3 Inappropriate Therapies

Inappropriate therapies (especially shocks) are one of the main issues to be avoided as they cause patient discomfort, are potentially proarrhythmic, and reduce battery life.

The two main causes of inappropriate shock are failure in discriminating SVA and signal misinterpretation.

Frequently SVA is associated with a fast ventricular response leading ventricular rate to fall into VT/VF detection zone causing inappropriate therapy release. This problem occurs more frequently with single-chamber ICDs that do not have atrial sensing capabilities. Dual-chamber devices can compare atrial and ventricular rates to set the origin of the. ICDs use a variety of algorithms to discriminate SVA from VT; major ones are listed below:

• *Atrioventricular rate comparison*: applies only in dual-chamber ICDs; when the ventricular rate is faster, the diagnosis is VT. When atrial and ventricular rates are equal, additional criteria are required for discrimination.
• *Onset*: useful for discrimination of gradually accelerating sinus tachycardia from sudden-onset VT. It applies when the RR interval shortens by a programmed percentage if compared with the average number of preceding beats. May fail in case of VT occurring during sinus tachycardia.
• *Stability*: useful for discrimination of fast response AF. It evaluates RR variability; when greater than a programmed percentage (e.g., 20 %), AF is supposed. It may fail in the case of very fast AF in which there is a pseudo-regularization of ventricular rate, in atrial flutter or in irregular VT.

- *Morphology*: it compares endocavitary electrocardiograms recorded during sinus rhythm and during VT. It is useful in single-chamber ICDs lacking of atrial information but may fail in intraventricular conduction delays and in rate-dependent conduction delays.
- *Rate duration*: it is an extreme lifesaving measure. It results in shock delivery after a programmable time interval even if the episode is classified as SVA; this algorithm is usually activated when there is a high risk of undertreatment of VT erroneously recognized as SVA, but it increases the risk of overtreatment.

Signal misinterpretation is the other big deal leading to inappropriate shocks. It may depend on some programmed variables; easily editable, external, and far-field interferences; or device/lead failure that usually requires an interventional approach. Main causes of signal misinterpretation are listed below:

- *T wave oversensing*: it happens when a high amplitude T wave is erroneously recognized as an R wave. It may happen because of the low ventricular sensing threshold necessary to recognize even low-amplitude VF. This problem can be solved by increasing sensing threshold, lengthening refractory period, or changing sensing decay parameters to suppress T wave detection.
- *Electromagnetic external interference*: external electromagnetic fields can be mistaken for intracardiac signals resulting in inappropriate arrhythmic detection and therapy. Common household appliances are not generally a problem, but some high-intensity fields such as high-voltage power lines, electric motors, magnetic resonance imaging, TENS units, electrocautery during surgery, neurostimulators, and radiotherapy should be avoided.
- *Myopotentials*: far-field myopotential recording may lead to inappropriate arrhythmic detection. This problem occurred in the past with unipolar leads using large sensing fields (from the lead tip to the generator case) and is now largely avoided with the modern bipolar leads, recording more localized signals only.
- *Lead failure*: lead fracture or insulation loss of continuity may cause external noise recording and inappropriate detection. In these cases lead extraction and/or new lead insertion is the only choice. Modern devices usually provide alerts for lead integrity.

12.2.4 Electrical Storm

12.2.4.1 Incidence and Clinical Predictors

Several studies examined the incidence of ES in ICD recipients, although ES definition was not standardized and the inclusion criteria and follow-up period were not homogeneous. Considering current definition, the incidence varies from 4 to 28 % in a follow-up period between 1 and 3 years [9]. In the sub-analysis of the AVID trial [10], including 499 patients treated for secondary prevention, the rate of ES was 20 % at 3-year follow-up. Of note, the incidence of ES in primary prevention trials appears lower (4 % in MADIT II), and in our experience [11], after a mean 2-year follow-up, only 13 patients (2 %) experienced an ICD treatment configuring an ES.

A recent meta-analysis [9] evaluated the real weight of ES as a risk factor and its clinical predictors. On the basis of 13 studies, a trend toward an increased prevalence of ES was associated with advanced age and male gender. Other factors related to ES in ICD carriers were heart failure-related clinical variables (as lower ejection fraction), an ICD implant for secondary prevention, the presence of monomorphic VT as triggering arrhythmias instead of polymorphic VTs and VF, and the treatment with class I antiarrhythmic drugs but not with amiodarone and beta-blockers. On the contrary, no significant differences between patients with ischemic or nonischemic dilated cardiomyopathy were reported. After meta-regression analysis, no significant interaction between any of the examined clinical variables and the increased risk of ES was confirmed.

The main clinical characteristics and clinical predictors of ES in the group of patients treated with a CRT-D have been considered in a multicenter experience including 631 patients, with a mean follow-up of 19 ± 11 months. In this study VT or VF episodes were detected and treated in 141 patients (22 %), and ES occurred in 45 (7 %). At univariate analysis, the only predictors of ES were the nonischemic etiology of cardiomyopathy and secondary prevention indication, while other common variables such as age, male gender, ejection fraction lower than 25 %, and advanced NYHA class did not correlate.

Our experience included 62 patients (mean age 66 years, 90 % male) admitted for ES during the period 2006–2012. The mean interval from implant to ES was 47 months. Ischemic heart disease was present in 30, nonischemic cardiomyopathy in 11, and other etiologies in 14, and 60 % of patients had been treated with ICD for secondary prevention. Mean ejection fraction was 35 %. In 23 patients the arrhythmia at admittance was incessant VT, while the remaining 39 experienced several VT/VF episodes, with a mean number of 6 shocks per patient. In more than half of patients (31), there wasn't a clear trigger and the ES rises from a primitive electrical instability. In the remaining the most frequent triggers were worsening heart failure, electrolyte imbalances, myocardial ischemia, and proarrhythmic drug side effects.

12.2.4.2 Prognosis

The majority of papers evaluating the role of ES as a mortality risk factor showed that it was associated with a threefold risk of death. ES maintained a significant value as risk factor even when compared with unclustered sustained VT/VF [9]. For the composite end point of all cause mortality, heart transplantation and hospitalization for heart failure ES was associated with a 3.39-fold increased risk.

The reported mortality among large series [12] of patients with ES treated by catheter ablation appeared extremely variable between 15 and 29 % during a follow-up ranging from 1 to 2.5 years. In our series, including patients treated not exclusively by catheter ablation, the overall survival of patients experiencing their first ES episode was 60 %, 50 %, and 44 % after 1, 2, and 3 years, respectively.

Considering that ES is associated with increased SCD and non-sudden cardiac mortality, Guerra et al. evaluated the association between ES and heart failure in patients with chronic heart failure and ICD. They reported that during 5-year follow-up, the survival estimates were not significantly different between patients with ES and HF worsening (36.4 vs. 38.5 months), while it was significantly lower in comparison to survival of patients with unclustered VT/VF episodes (49.2 months). The primary mortality cause in ES group was refractory heart failure (59 %), followed by noncardiac conditions and by SCD in only two patients. Even hospitalization-free rate was lower in both ES and HF worsening groups in comparison to patients with unclustered VT/VF episodes (15.4 vs. 20.1 vs. 36.1 months), while the hospitalization rates were not significantly different between ES and HF worsening groups. The conclusions of the authors were that heart failure patients admitted for ES show important outcome analogies with patients admitted for acute heart failure and that ES should be identified as an important clinical consequence of heart failure decompensation.

12.3   What the Cardiologist Should Know

ES is a medical emergency potentially leading to acute cardiac failure and cardiogenic shock and requiring a multidisciplinary approach.

Initial diagnostic workup includes physical examination, electrocardiogram (ECG), chest X-ray, echocardiogram, blood gas analysis, electrolytes, serum creatinine evaluation, and ICD interrogation.

The first issue to assess in a patient with multiple ICD shocks is to seek ICD intervention causes.

In case of appropriate therapies due to VT/VF, it is necessary first of all to rule out reversible causes of ES including electrolyte imbalances, acute ischemia, worsening heart failure, infective state, hyperthyroidism, and proarrhythmic drugs. In a large series reversible causes of ES account for no more than 10 % of cases referred to EP labs [4].

Following initial evaluation, an accurate patient's risk stratification should be made according to hemodynamic tolerance of the clinical VT and comorbidities [13]. Hemodynamic decompensation defined as sustained hypotension (i.e., systolic blood pressure <80–90 mmHg) despite increasing doses of vasopressors and requiring mechanical hemodynamic support (i.e., intra-aortic balloon pump, left ventricular assist devices, or extracorporeal membrane oxygenation) [14] makes the patient at high risk by itself and in some cases even at the temporary restoration of sinus rhythm. In case of hemodynamically tolerated VT, the presence of at least one comorbidity such as left ventricular ejection fraction less than 30 %, serum creatinine level >1.5 mg/dl, chronic occlusion of left anterior descending coronary artery, and severe chronic lung disease makes the patient particularly high risk [13]. All high-risk patients should be admitted to intensive care unit (ICU) and, if necessary, undergo circulatory and/or ventilatory support and/or hemodialysis.

All the efforts should be made to reduce VT/VF episodes to avoid further shocks considering even in combination of a complex strategic approach including antiarrhythmic drug therapy, device reprogramming, deep sedation/mechanical assistance, and catheter ablation.

12.3.1 Antiarrhythmic Drugs

Initial treatment of ES usually involves the use of antiarrhythmic drugs, weighing their proarrhythmic risk and negative inotropic effect, to prevent arrhythmic recurrences.

The cornerstone of antiarrhythmic therapy still remains sympathetic blockade with *beta-blockers* to suppress the adrenergic drive to VT recurrence [15]. Although all beta-blockers are able to reduce susceptibility to VT/VF as class action, most of the studies analyzed *propranolol*. In patients with HF, propranolol resulted to be more effective than *metoprolol* in reducing sympathetic tone due to its capability of blocking both $\beta1$ and $\beta2$ receptors and to its lipophilic nature that enables penetration within the central nervous system blocking also presynaptic adrenergic receptors [16, 17]. Sympathetic blockade is able not only to suppress ES [18] but also to improve short-term survival more than the combined antiarrhythmic therapy with lidocaine, procainamide, and bretylium [15]. In severely compromised patients, intravenous short-acting drugs like *esmolol* should be preferred [19]. The first-choice antiarrhythmic drug should be *amiodarone*, even in combination with propranolol that effectively controlled ES and improved survival [15, 18]. When amiodarone is administered intravenously, it reduces adrenergic tone, blocks sodium and L-calcium channels without prolonging ventricular refractoriness, and, when administered, orally prolongs ventricular refractory period [20, 21]. When ineffective alone or in combination with beta-blockers, amiodarone may be helpful even in adjunct to other agents [22]. Even patients who previously keep amiodarone may beneficiate from a reloading dose/therapy adjustment if serum levels of amiodarone/desethil-amiodarone are under therapeutic levels. The acute administration is relatively safe even in patients with depressed ejection fraction due to its low inotropic negative effect. It can increase the defibrillation threshold, making potentially ineffective ICD therapy; consequently ICD defibrillation energy should be re-tested or re-evaluated. Long-term amiodarone assumption is burdened by several side effects like thyroid, liver, and lung toxicity, sometimes forcing to therapy discontinuation. In case of amiodarone failure, other additionally drugs may be considered such as procainamide both orally or intravenously. The use of multiple antiarrhythmic drugs makes the drug-to-drug interaction unpredictable, potentially increasing the side effect occurrence. The use of *lidocaine* is limited by its relatively incapacity to terminate scar-related VT [23]. Lidocaine is a sodium rapid channel blocker that binds to channels in a use-dependent way. During ischemic VT, the altered membrane potential as the pH reduction [24] increases the rate of drug binding, making lidocaine effective in terminating arrhythmias. The pharmacodynamic proprieties make lidocaine not so effective in settings different from ischemic arrhythmias, maintaining a role only for the treatment of polymorphic VT associated with ischemia (IIb recommendation according to the American College of Cardiology/ American Heart Association guidelines [25]).

Procainamide (not available in all countries) is another IC class antiarrhythmic drug commonly used as second- or third- line therapy in refractory VTs. Procainamide acts as fast sodium channel blocker, while its active metabolite N-acetylprocainamide blocks potassium channels and accounts for much of the antiarrhythmic effect in vivo as well as side effects like QT interval prolongation. Care must be taken in administering the drug in patients with low ejection fraction due to the high risk of hypotension.

12.3.2 Device Reprogramming

Several studies demonstrated that repeated ICD shocks are associated with increased mortality as well as with a reduction of quality of life [10]. For these reasons optimization of ICD programming in order to avoid unnecessary shock is mandatory in patients experiencing ES. As stated above, arrhythmic detection and treatment by ICD is a step process including several variables such as heart rate threshold, number of intervals to detect, discrimination of SVA, and type and number of therapies released. Each of these steps can be tailored upon patient characteristics to avoid unnecessary treatment.

12.3.2.1 Higher Heart Rate Threshold

Usually patients treated with ICD for primary prevention tend to develop fast VT, while patients treated for secondary prevention usually have slower VT with a wider overlap with SVA [26]. On this basis, the first may benefit from higher rate detection zones, while the latter needs slower rate detection zones and improved SVA discriminating algorithms. Even better, rate detection zones can be tailored upon patient's clinical history when previous arrhythmia episodes occurred. In three trials (PREPARE, MADIT-RIT, and PROVIDE), higher rate detection zones demonstrated reduce ICD shocks without increasing both syncope and death risk.

12.3.2.2 Longer Detection Period

The effect of prolonging arrhythmic detection time is well studied especially in the primary prevention setting with lower data available in the setting of secondary prevention.

The REVELANT study showed that a higher number of intervals for arrhythmic detection (30/40 vs. 12/16) significantly reduced the incidence of ICD intervention without increasing syncope or death in patients with ICD for primary prevention and nonischemic cardiomyopathy. MADIT-RIT trial showed a reduction of both inappropriate therapy and all-cause mortality with a 60-s delay at 170–199 bpm, a

12-s delay at 200–249 bpm, and a 2.5-s delay at ≥250 bpm vs. conventional programming. These results were recently confirmed by ADVANCE III trial [27] in which the combination of a higher number of intervals to detection (30/40 vs. 18/24) with ATP therapy during charge significantly reduced either appropriate or inappropriate therapies regardless of ICD type and indication. Even in the PROVIDE trial, multi-parametric programming including higher detection rate, longer detection intervals, and optimized SVA discriminating algorithms was associated with better overall survival and reduction of ICD shocks without increasing arrhythmic syncope risk, and the PainFree SST trial confirmed that longer detection intervals are safe in terms of risk of syncope. Of all these studies, only ADVANCE III and the PainFree SST included patients with both primary and secondary preventions for ICD, while the remaining trials focused only on patients treated for primary prevention.

12.3.2.3 Improving ATP Programming

ATP therapy demonstrated to be highly effective in terminating VTs, reducing unnecessary shocks and consequently improving survival, quality of life, and generator life. In several studies 85–90 % of "slow" VTs (<188–200 bpm) [28] and 54–72 % of "fast" VTs (188–250 bpm) [29, 27] were terminated by ATP. As stated before, ATP therapy can be administered as *bursts or ramps* on the basis of the pacing cycle length variations. Bursts and ramps proved similar efficacy in treating slower VTs [28], while fast VTs (>200 bpm) were best treated by bursts that also showed a lower risk of arrhythmic acceleration than ramps. Due to less efficacy of ATP in terminating fast VTs (>200 bpm) and the negative hemodynamic consequences of such arrhythmias, usually in the fast VT and VF zone, *ATP is delivered during capacitor charge* to avoid any delay in shock therapy. The majority of VTs were effectively interrupted by one or two ATP attempts with only a minority of patients responsive to more than three attempts [30, 31], and for this reason programming more than three ATP attempts should be discouraged. In CRT-D recipients, biventricular ATP should be preferred to right ventricular ATP due to its higher efficacy and safety [32, 33]. The last key point in ATP programming is burst cycle length that can be empirically programmed at 85–90 % of the arrhythmic cycle length for fast VTs and at 70–80 % for slower ones. When ATP appears ineffective in VT termination, the analysis of the post pacing interval can allow tailoring ATP programming upon patient characteristics, for example, by shortening drive cycle length or by increasing the number of paced beats [34].

Accordingly to all these data, the increase of detection time and threshold rate in patients experiencing ES helps to prevent both inappropriate and unnecessary shocks, making ICD reprogramming a mandatory step in the clinical workup of ES.

In case of inappropriate therapies, specific measures must be taken: e.g., change ICD detection parameters, enhance drug therapy, or consider catheter ablation in case of SVA; temporarily turn off the device before lead replacement in case of lead fracture/failure.

12.3.3 Sedation, General Anesthesia/Mechanical Ventilation, and Mechanical Hemodynamic Support

The sympathetic adrenergic activation in patients experiencing multiple shocks due to ES may perpetuate VT/VF [35] and render the arrhythmias life threatening and refractory to several maneuvers. Therefore, some patients with ES should be sedated or even undergo general anesthesia to reduce sympathetic tone and suppress ventricular electrical instability. *Propofol* has been reported to suppress ES [36, 37], but this beneficial effect may be offset by the inotropic negative effect. In this regard, only few data are available in literature about the effect of deep sedation/general anesthesia on the prognosis of ES patients, and most of them are extrapolated from patients undergoing catheter ablation to treat ES. Drugs inducing general anesthesia should be considered with attention because they can exacerbate hypotension and depress cardiac function [14]. Deep sedation with *remifentanil* even in association with a *benzodiazepine* like midazolam should be preferred as it is able to reduce sympathetic hypertone and provide analgesia avoiding dangerous negative inotropic effects [38–40]. A valuable alternative may be *dexmedetomidine* [41], an α2 presynaptic adrenergic receptor agonist able to markedly reduce sympathetic tone by both enhancing central vagal tone [42] and inhibiting presynaptical adrenaline release [43]. However, it has important side effects like hypotension and bradycardia [44] that should be rigorously monitored during its usage.

General anesthesia and mechanical ventilation should be reserved only to patients with hemodynamically non-tolerated arrhythmias refractory to all therapies. Such patients may benefit from hemodynamic mechanical support like *intra-aortic-balloon pump* (IABP), *left ventricular assistance devices* such as the Impella (Abiomed Inc., Danvers, MA) [45–47], and even *extracorporeal membrane oxygenation* (ECMO) [48, 49]. These devices can not only suppress ischemic VTs by increasing coronary perfusion but can be effective in suppressing ES reducing LV afterload and wall tension [50] as well as prevent multiple organ failure sustaining organ perfusion. Last but not least, they have a key role in mapping and ablating unstable VTs. Some patients experiencing refractory unstable arrhythmias should also be carefully evaluated for urgent check for cardiac transplantation.

12.3.4 Neuraxial Modulation (Thoracic Epidural Anesthesia, Cardiac Sympathetic Denervation)

Given the importance of the autonomic nervous system in triggering and maintaining ventricular arrhythmias, sympathetic neuromodulation through thoracic epidural anesthesia [51], cardiac sympathetic denervation (CSD), and spinal cord stimulation may help in reducing arrhythmic burden in selected patient with ES refractory to multiple antiarrhythmic drugs and catheter ablation. CSD is usually performed via video-assisted thoracic surgery and consists of removal the lower third of the stellate ganglia (to avoid Claude-Bernard-Horner syndrome) as well as T2–T4 thoracic ganglia. The resection is usually performed on the left side, reserving bilateral CSD for selected cases. The procedure should be performed in referral centers only, due to special anesthesiology skills required such as selective bronchus intubation management. Most of what we know about the results of the procedure results from case reports [52, 51, 53], but in a prospective study of 41 patients with ES refractory to medical therapy and catheter ablation, CDS demonstrated to be effective in prolonging ICD shock-free survival at 1-year follow-up with greater effect of bilateral CDS compared to left CDS only [54].

12.3.5 Catheter Ablation

Currently, radiofrequency catheter (RF) ablation represents the mainstay treatment of recurrent VTs and even of ES. Several studies demonstrated how catheter ablation may prevent VT recurrence as well as improve survival of ES patients with a growing effectiveness due to technological improvement and deeper knowledge of arrhythmogenic substrate [14]. In the past, RF ablation was considered as the last chance treatment in patients refractory to multiple antiarrhythmic drugs, but in the last decade there has been a growing evidence for early referral to RF ablation in case of recurrent ICD therapies or even prophylactically [55–57]. RF ablation showed to be highly effective in suppressing refractory VTs in the acute management of ES, reaching an acute success rate of 80 % in the largest series [40, 12, 58, 59], especially when the end point of non-inducibility of all clinical VTs was reached [12]. As stated before, patients with unstable hemodynamic VTs should be referred for mechanical assistance in order to allow mapping and ablation but also those with apparently stable arrhythmia may develop acute hemodynamic decompensation during RF ablation procedure. In a preliminary study, a simple score named PAINESD taking in account patient's baseline comorbidities (Pulmonary chronic obstructive disease, Age older than 60, Ischemic cardiomyopathy, NYHA class III or IV, Ejection fraction lower than 25 %, Storm at presentation, and Diabetes mellitus) was tested to predict acute decompensation during VT catheter ablation in order to select patients who may benefit prophylactic mechanical support [14] (Fig. 12.1).

12.4 Indication for Follow-Up and Referral

All patients who experienced an ES episode remain at high risk of recurrences even if effectively treated with catheter ablation and multiple antiarrhythmic drug prophylaxis. Often ES is the expression of worsening of the underling heart disease. For these reasons all patients who developed at least one episode of ES

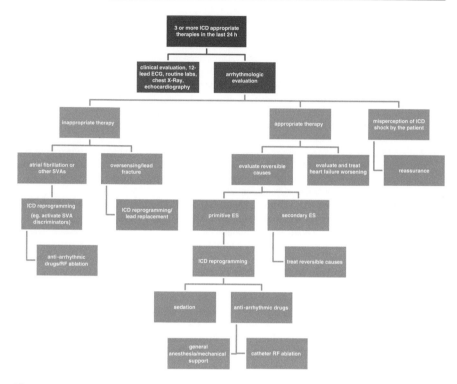

Fig. 12.1 A suggested algorithm/pathway for diagnosis and treatment of ES

should be referred both to a heart failure specialist and proper electrophysiological management in order to optimize the heart failure therapy and evaluate indication to heart transplantation or left ventricular assistance devices both as a bridge to transplant and as destination therapy. Arrhythmic follow-up may be best done with home monitoring of the ICD that allows a prompt evaluation of arrhythmic events.

References

1. Pedersen CT, Kay GN, Kalman J, Borggrefe M, Della-Bella P, Dickfeld T, Dorian P, Huikuri H, Kim Y-H, Knight B, Marchlinski F, Ross D, Sacher F, Sapp J, Shivkumar K, Soejima K, Tada H, Alexander ME, Triedman JK, Yamada T, Kirchhof P, Lip GYH, Kuck KH, Mont L, Haines D, Indik J, Dimarco J, Exner D, Iesaka Y, Savelieva I, EP-Europace, UK. EHRA/HRS/ APHRS expert consensus on ventricular arrhythmias. Heart Rhythm. 2014;11:e166–96.
2. McMurray JJV, Adamopoulos S, Anker SD, Auricchio A, Böhm M, Dickstein K, Falk V, Filippatos G, Fonseca C, Gomez-Sanchez MA, Jaarsma T, Køber L, Lip GYH, Maggioni AP, Parkhomenko A, Pieske BM, Popescu BA, Rønnevik PK, Rutten FH, Schwitter J, Seferovic P,

Stepinska J, Trindade PT, Voors AA, Zannad F, Zeiher A, ESC Committee for Practice Guidelines. ESC Guidelines for the diagnosis and treatment of acute and chronic heart failure 2012: The Task Force for the Diagnosis and Treatment of Acute and Chronic Heart Failure 2012 of the European Society of Cardiology. Developed in collaboration with the Heart Failure Association (HFA) of the ESC. Eur Heart J. 2012;33:1787–847.

3. Mosterd A, Hoes AW. Clinical epidemiology of heart failure. Heart. 2007;93:1137–46.
4. Hohnloser SH, Al-Khalidi HR, Pratt CM, Brum JM, Tatla DS, Tchou P, Dorian P, SHock Inhibition Evaluation with AzimiLiDe (SHIELD) Investigators. Electrical storm in patients with an implantable defibrillator: incidence, features, and preventive therapy: insights from a randomized trial. Eur Heart J. 2006;27:3027–32.
5. Wathen MS. Prospective randomized multicenter trial of empirical antitachycardia pacing versus shocks for spontaneous rapid ventricular tachycardia in patients with implantable cardioverter-defibrillators: Pacing Fast Ventricular Tachycardia Reduces Shock Therapies (PainFREE Rx II) trial results. Circulation. 2004;110:2591–6.
6. Wilkoff BL, Williamson BD, Stern RS, Moore SL, Lu F, Lee SW, Birgersdotter-Green UM, Wathen MS, Van Gelder IC, Heubner BM, Brown ML, Holloman KK. Strategic programming of detection and therapy parameters in implantable cardioverter-defibrillators reduces shocks in primary prevention patients. J Am Coll Cardiol. 2008;52:541–50.
7. Wilkoff BL, Ousdigian KT, Sterns LD, Wang ZJ, Wilson RD, Morgan JM. A comparison of empiric to physician-tailored programming of implantable cardioverter-defibrillators. J Am Coll Cardiol. 2006;48:330–9.
8. Gunderson BD, Abeyratne AI, Olson WH, Swerdlow CD. Effect of programmed number of intervals to detect ventricular fibrillation on implantable cardioverter-defibrillator aborted and unnecessary shocks. Pacing Clin Electrophysiol. 2007;30:157–65.
9. Guerra F, Shkoza M, Scappini L, Flori M, Capucci A. Role of electrical storm as a mortality and morbidity risk factor and its clinical predictors: a meta-analysis. Europace. 2014;16:347–53.
10. Tan VH, Wilton SB, Kuriachan V, Sumner GL, Exner DV. Impact of programming strategies aimed at reducing nonessential implantable cardioverter defibrillator therapies on mortality: a systematic review and meta-analysis. Circ Arrhythm Electrophysiol. 2014;7:164–70.
11. Proclemer A, Muser D, Campana A, Zoni-Berisso M, Zecchin M, Locatelli A, Brieda M, Gramegna L, Santarone M, Chiodi L, Mazzone P, Rebellato L, Facchin D. Indication to cardioverter-defibrillator therapy and outcome in real world primary prevention. Data from the IRIDE [Italian registry of prophylactic implantation of defibrillators] study. Int J Cardiol. 2013;168:1416–21.
12. Carbucicchio C, Santamaria M, Trevisi N, Maccabelli G, Giraldi F, Fassini G, Riva S, Moltrasio M, Cireddu M, Veglia F, Della Bella P. Catheter ablation for the treatment of electrical storm in patients with implantable cardioverter-defibrillators: short- and long-term outcomes in a prospective single-center study. Circulation. 2008;117:462–9.
13. Bella PD, Baratto F, Tsiachris D, Trevisi N, Vergara P, Bisceglia C, Petracca F, Carbucicchio C, Benussi S, Maisano F, Alfieri O, Pappalardo F, Zangrillo A, Maccabelli G. Management of ventricular tachycardia in the setting of a dedicated unit for the treatment of complex ventricular arrhythmias: long-term outcome after ablation. Circulation. 2013;127:1359–68.
14. Santangeli P, Muser D, Zado ES, Magnani S, Khetpal S, Hutchinson MD, Supple G, Frankel DS, Garcia FC, Bala R, Riley MP, Lin D, Rame JE, Schaller R, Dixit S, Marchlinski FE, Callans DJ. Acute hemodynamic decompensation during catheter ablation of scar-related VT: incidence, predictors and impact on mortality. Circ Arrhythm Electrophysiol. 2015;8:68–75.
15. Nademanee K, Taylor R, Bailey WE, Rieders DE, Kosar EM. Treating electrical storm: sympathetic blockade versus advanced cardiac life support-guided therapy. Circulation. 2000;102:742–7.
16. Bristow MR, Ginsburg R, Umans V, Fowler M, Minobe W, Rasmussen R, Zera P, Menlove R, Shah P, Jamieson S. Beta 1-and beta 2-adrenergic-receptor subpopulations in nonfailing and failing human ventricular myocardium: coupling of both receptor subtypes to muscle contraction and selective beta 1-receptor down-regulation in heart failure. Circ Res. 1986;59:297–309.

17. Billman GE, Castillo LC, Hensley J, Hohl CM, Altschuld RA. Beta2-adrenergic receptor antagonists protect against ventricular fibrillation: in vivo and in vitro evidence for enhanced sensitivity to beta2-adrenergic stimulation in animals susceptible to sudden death. Circulation. 1997;96:1914–22.
18. Tsagalou EP, Kanakakis J, Rokas S, Anastasiou-Nana MI. Suppression by propranolol and amiodarone of an electrical storm refractory to metoprolol and amiodarone. Int J Cardiol. 2005;99:341–2.
19. Brodine WN, Tung RT, Lee JK, Hockstad ES, Moss AJ, Zareba W, Hall WJ, Andrews M, McNitt S, Daubert JP. Effects of beta-blockers on implantable cardioverter defibrillator therapy and survival in the patients with ischemic cardiomyopathy (from the Multicenter Automatic Defibrillator Implantation Trial-II). Am J Cardiol. 2005;96:691–5.
20. Kodama I, Kamiya K, Honjo H, Toyama J. Acute and chronic effects of amiodarone on mammalian ventricular cells. Jpn Heart J. 1996;37:719–30.
21. Du XJ, Esler MD, Dart AM. Sympatholytic action of intravenous amiodarone in the rat heart. Circulation. 1995;91:462–70.
22. Vassallo P, Trohman RG. Prescribing amiodarone: an evidence-based review of clinical indications. JAMA. 2007;298:1312–22.
23. Guidelines 2000 for Cardiopulmonary Resuscitation and Emergency Cardiovascular Care. Part 6: advanced cardiovascular life support: section 5: pharmacology I: agents for arrhythmias. The American Heart Association in collaboration with the International Liaison Committee on Resuscitation. Circulation. 2000;102:I112–28.
24. Nasir N, Taylor A, Doyle TK, Pacifico A. Evaluation of intravenous lidocaine for the termination of sustained monomorphic ventricular tachycardia in patients with coronary artery disease with or without healed myocardial infarction. Am J Cardiol. 1994;74:1183–6.
25. American College of Cardiology, American Heart Association Task Force, European Society of Cardiology Committee for Practice Guidelines, European Heart Rhythm Association, Heart Rhythm Society, Zipes DP, Camm AJ, Borggrefe M, Buxton AE, Chaitman B, Fromer M, Gregoratos G, Klein G, Moss AJ, Myerburg RJ, Priori SG, Quinones MA, Roden DM, Silka MJ, Tracy C, Smith SC, Jacobs AK, Adams CD, Antman EM, Anderson JL, Hunt SA, Halperin JL, Nishimura R, Ornato JP, Page RL, Riegel B, Priori SG, Blanc J-J, Budaj A, Camm AJ, Dean V, Deckers JW, Despres C, Dickstein K, Lekakis J, McGregor K, Metra M, Morais J, Osterspey A, Tamargo JL, Zamorano JL. ACC/AHA/ESC 2006 guidelines for management of patients with ventricular arrhythmias and the prevention of sudden cardiac death: a report of the American College of Cardiology/American Heart Association Task Force and the European Society of Cardiology Committee for Practice Guidelines (writing committee to develop Guidelines for Management of Patients With Ventricular Arrhythmias and the Prevention of Sudden Cardiac Death). J Am Coll Cardiol. 2006;48:e247–346.
26. Wilkoff BL, Hess M, Young J, Abraham WT. Differences in tachyarrhythmia detection and implantable cardioverter defibrillator therapy by primary or secondary prevention indication in cardiac resynchronization therapy patients. J Cardiovasc Electrophysiol. 2004;15:1002–9.
27. Gasparini M, Proclemer A, Klersy C, Kloppe A, Lunati M, Ferrer JBM, Hersi A, Gulaj M, Wijfels MCEF, Santi E, Manotta L, Arenal A. Effect of long-detection interval vs standard-detection interval for implantable cardioverter-defibrillators on antitachycardia pacing and shock delivery: the ADVANCE III randomized clinical trial. JAMA. 2013;309:1903–11.
28. Sweeney MO. Antitachycardia pacing for ventricular tachycardia using implantable cardioverter defibrillators. Pacing Clin Electrophysiol. 2004;27:1292–305.
29. Wathen MS, DeGroot PJ, Sweeney MO, Stark AJ, Otterness MF, Adkisson WO, Canby RC, Khalighi K, Machado C, Rubenstein DS, Volosin KJ, PainFREE Rx II Investigators. Prospective randomized multicenter trial of empirical antitachycardia pacing versus shocks for spontaneous rapid ventricular tachycardia in patients with implantable cardioverter-defibrillators: Pacing Fast Ventricular Tachycardia Reduces Shock Therapies (PainFREE Rx II) trial results. Circulation. 2004;110:2591–6.
30. Martins RP, Blangy H, Muresan L, Freysz L, Groben L, Zinzius P-Y, Schwartz J, Sellal J-M, Aliot E, Sadoul N. Safety and efficacy of programming a high number of antitachycardia pacing attempts for fast ventricular tachycardia: a prospective study. Europace. 2012;14:1457–64.

31. Anguera I, Dallaglio P, Sabaté X, Nuñez E, Gracida M, Di Marco A, Sugrañes G, Cequier A. The benefit of a second burst antitachycardia sequence for fast ventricular tachycardia in patients with implantable cardioverter defibrillators. Pacing Clin Electrophysiol. 2014;37:486–94.
32. Haghjoo M, Hajahmadi M, Fazelifar AF, Sadr-Ameli MA. Efficacy and safety of different antitachycardia pacing sites in the termination of ventricular tachycardia in patients with biventricular implantable cardioverter-defibrillator. Europace. 2011;13:509–13.
33. Gasparini M, Anselme F, Clementy J, Santini M, Martínez-Ferrer J, De Santo T, Santi E, Schwab JO, ADVANCE CRT-D Investigators. BIVentricular versus right ventricular antitachy-cardia pacing to terminate ventricular tachyarrhythmias in patients receiving cardiac resyn-chronization therapy: the ADVANCE CRT-D Trial. Am Heart J. 2010;159:1116–1123.e2.
34. Madhavan M, Friedman PA. Optimal programming of implantable cardiac-defibrillators. Circulation. 2013;128:659–72.
35. Zipes DP, Barber MJ, Takahashi N, Gilmour RF. Influence of the autonomic nervous system on the genesis of cardiac arrhythmias. Pacing Clin Electrophysiol. 1983;6:1210–20.
36. Mulpuru SK, Patel DV, Wilbur SL, Vasavada BC, Furqan T. Electrical storm and termination with propofol therapy: a case report. Int J Cardiol. 2008;128:e6–8.
37. Burjorjee JE, Milne B. Propofol for electrical storm; a case report of cardioversion and sup-pression of ventricular tachycardia by propofol. Can J Anaesth. 2002;49:973–7.
38. Ogletree ML, Sprung J, Moravec CS. Effects of remifentanil on the contractility of failing human heart muscle. J Cardiothorac Vasc Anesth. 2005;19:763–7.
39. Mandel JE, Hutchinson MD, Marchlinski FE. Remifentanil-midazolam sedation provides hemodynamic stability and comfort during epicardial ablation of ventricular tachycardia. J Cardiovasc Electrophysiol. 2011;22:464–6.
40. Brugada J, Berruezo A, Cuesta A, Osca J, Chueca E, Fosch X, Wayar L, Mont L. Nonsurgical transthoracic epicardial radiofrequency ablation: an alternative in incessant ventricular tachy-cardia. J Am Coll Cardiol. 2003;41:2036–43.
41. Tarvainen MP, Georgiadis S, Laitio T, Lipponen JA, Karjalainen PA, Kaskinoro K, Scheinin H. Heart rate variability dynamics during low-dose propofol and dexmedetomidine anesthesia. Ann Biomed Eng. 2012;40:1802–13.
42. Kamibayashi T, Hayashi Y, Mammoto T, Yamatodani A, Sumikawa K, Yoshiya I. Role of the vagus nerve in the antidysrhythmic effect of dexmedetomidine on halothane/epinephrine dys-rhythmias in dogs. Anesthesiology. 1995;83:992–9.
43. Hayashi Y, Sumikawa K, Maze M, Yamatodani A, Kamibayashi T, Kuro M, Yoshiya I. Dexmedetomidine prevents epinephrine-induced arrhythmias through stimulation of central alpha 2 adrenoceptors in halothane-anesthetized dogs. Anesthesiology. 1991;75:113–7.
44. Gerlach AT, Murphy CV. Dexmedetomidine-associated bradycardia progressing to pulseless electrical activity: case report and review of the literature. Pharmacotherapy. 2009;29:1492.
45. Miller MA, Dukkipati SR, Mittnacht AJ, Chinitz JS, Belliveau L, Koruth JS, Gomes JA, d' Avila A, Reddy VY. Activation and entrainment mapping of hemodynamically unstable ven-tricular tachycardia using a percutaneous left ventricular assist device. J Am Coll Cardiol. 2011;58:1363–71.
46. Abuissa H, Roshan J, Lim B, Asirvatham SJ. Use of the Impella microaxial blood pump for ablation of hemodynamically unstable ventricular tachycardia. J Cardiovasc Electrophysiol. 2010;21:458–61.
47. Miller MA, Dukkipati SR, Chinitz JS, Koruth JS, Mittnacht AJ, Napolitano C, d' Avila A, Reddy VY. Percutaneous hemodynamic support with Impella 2.5 during scar-related ventricu-lar tachycardia ablation (PERMIT 1). Circ Arrhythm Electrophysiol. 2013;6:151–9.
48. Ücer E, Fredersdorf S, Jungbauer C, Debl K, Philipp A, Amann M, Holzamer A, Keyser A, Hilker M, Luchner A, Schmid C, Riegger G, Endemann D. A unique access for the ablation catheter to treat electrical storm in a patient with extracorporeal life support. Europace. 2014;16:299–302.
49. Lü F, Eckman PM, Liao KK, Apostolidou I, John R, Chen T, Das GS, Francis GS, Lei H, Trohman RG, Benditt DG. Catheter ablation of hemodynamically unstable ventricular tachy-cardia with mechanical circulatory support. Int J Cardiol. 2013;168:3859–65.

50. Franz MR, Burkhoff D, Yue DT, Sagawa K. Mechanically induced action potential changes and arrhythmia in isolated and in situ canine hearts. Cardiovasc Res. 1989;23:213–23.
51. Bourke T, Vaseghi M, Michowitz Y, Sankhla V, Shah M, Swapna N, Boyle NG, Mahajan A, Narasimhan C, Lokhandwala Y, Shivkumar K. Neuraxial modulation for refractory ventricular arrhythmias: value of thoracic epidural anesthesia and surgical left cardiac sympathetic denervation. Circulation. 2010;121:2255–62.
52. Ajijola OA, Lellouche N, Bourke T, Tung R, Ahn S, Mahajan A, Shivkumar K. Bilateral cardiac sympathetic denervation for the management of electrical storm. J Am Coll Cardiol. 2012;59:91–2.
53. Estes EH, Izlar HL. Recurrent ventricular tachycardia. A case successfully treated by bilateral cardiac sympathectomy. Am J Med. 1961;31:493–7.
54. Vaseghi M, Gima J, Kanaan C, Ajijola OA, Marmureanu A, Mahajan A, Shivkumar K. Cardiac sympathetic denervation in patients with refractory ventricular arrhythmias or electrical storm: intermediate and long-term follow-up. Heart Rhythm. 2014;11:360–6.
55. Stevenson WG, Wilber DJ, Natale A, Jackman WM, Marchlinski FE, Talbert T, Gonzalez MD, Worley SJ, Daoud EG, Hwang C, Schuger C, Bump TE, Jazayeri M, Tomassoni GF, Kopelman HA, Soejima K, Nakagawa H, Multicenter Thermocool VT Ablation Trial Investigators. Irrigated radiofrequency catheter ablation guided by electroanatomic mapping for recurrent ventricular tachycardia after myocardial infarction: the multicenter thermocool ventricular tachycardia ablation trial. Circulation. 2008;118:2773–82.
56. Reddy VY, Reynolds MR, Neuzil P, Richardson AW, Taborsky M, Jongnarangsin K, Kralovec S, Sediva L, Ruskin JN, Josephson ME. Prophylactic catheter ablation for the prevention of defibrillator therapy. N Engl J Med. 2007;357:2657–65.
57. Kuck K-H, Schaumann A, Eckardt L, Willems S, Ventura R, Delacrétaz E, Pitschner H-F, Kautzner J, Schumacher B, Hansen PS, VTACH study group. Catheter ablation of stable ventricular tachycardia before defibrillator implantation in patients with coronary heart disease (VTACH): a multicentre randomised controlled trial. Lancet. 2010;375:31–40.
58. Silva RMFL, Mont L, Nava S, Rojel U, Matas M, Brugada J. Radiofrequency catheter ablation for arrhythmic storm in patients with an implantable cardioverter defibrillator. Pacing Clin Electrophysiol. 2004;27:971–5.
59. Strickberger SA, Man KC, Daoud EG, Goyal R, Brinkman K, Hasse C, Bogun F, Knight BP, Weiss R, Bahu M, Morady F. A prospective evaluation of catheter ablation of ventricular tachycardia as adjuvant therapy in patients with coronary artery disease and an implantable cardioverter-defibrillator. Circulation. 1997;96:1525–31.

Emergency Surgery and Cardiac Devices 13

Massimo Zecchin, Luigi Rivetti, Gianfranco Sinagra,
Marco Merlo, and Aneta Aleksova

13.1 Focusing on the Issue

The number of patients with CIED (Cardiac Implantable Electric Devices) who need emergency surgery has been increasing in the last decades, considering the spread of ICD (Implantable Cardiovetrer-Defibrillator) and CRT (Cardiac Resynchronization Therapy) implantations for sudden death prevention and heart failure treatment.

It is estimated that about three million patients worldwide have a pacemaker (PM) and about 500,000 patients have an ICD [1]. According to EUCOMED data, in Europe nearly 1000 PM and 170 ICD new implantations were performed every million inhabitants in 2012. Although the implant rate of PMs has not significantly changed, there has been an increase of ICD and CRT implantations in the last decade, after the publication of several trials proving their efficacy. Despite some regional differences, this trend can be observed in most western countries.

In case of urgent surgical intervention, patients with CIED (especially ICD) can be considered at high risk for many reasons, mostly due to the underlying cardiac disease, hemodynamic impairment/left ventricular dysfunction (in particular those with ICDs), and the advanced age (in particular those with PMs) [2].

In addition, during surgical interventions, transient or even permanent malfunctions of the device, because of electromagnetic interferences or mechanical damages, are possible [3].

M. Zecchin (✉) • G. Sinagra • M. Merlo • A. Aleksova
Cardiovascular Department, Ospedali Riuniti and University of Trieste, Trieste, Italy
e-mail: massimo.zecchin@alice.it

L. Rivetti
Department of Clinical and Experimental Medicine, University of Messina,
Messina, Italy
e-mail: dott.luigirivetti@virgilio.it

© Springer International Publishing Switzerland 2016
M. Zecchin, G. Sinagra (eds.), *The Arrhythmic Patient in the Emergency Department: A Practical Guide for Cardiologists and Emergency Physicians*,
DOI 10.1007/978-3-319-24328-3_13

Electromagnetic fields can potentially cause several malfunctions: damage to the CIED circuitry, pacemaker inhibition, noise tracking, asynchronous pacing, communication failure, etc. [4].

An electromagnetic field is characterized by a wavelength, a frequency, and a field strength. The range of frequency emitted by sources such as magnetic resonance imaging (MRI) and electrosurgery is between 0 Hz and 450 MHz. The electric field strength is measured in volts per meter, while the magnetic field intensity components of electromagnetic fields are measured in amperes per meter. Electromagnetic field energy decreases as an inverse squared function of distance from the source, so the risk of exposure is fourfold lower just doubling the distance from the source.

Even static magnetic fields can be a possible cause of CIED malfunction; sterile magnetic drapes, frequently used during surgery to hold metal instruments, can potentially interfere with the function of PM and ICDs if positioned at a distance less than 15 cm [5].

Electrocautery is associated with tissue heating. However, conductive devices and leads, particularly when placed in a loop configuration, can increase the risk of burns due to the inductive heating of the lead conductor from radiofrequency fields.

In recent years, a great effort to minimize CIED has been performed. Generators are shielded by hermetically sealed titanium or stainless steel cases. The extent of shielding varies depending on the manufacturer, weight of the device, and dimensions and usually rejects electric fields >2 MHz.

EMI are also reduced by the use of bipolar sensing and low-pass filters. However, frequencies between 0 and 60 Hz overlaps the cardiac signal range so a "noise reversion feature" is activated when signals are detected in the noise-sampling period of the atrial and ventricular refractory periods, programming the device in asynchronous pacing.

Additionally, lead design was modified to improve shielding from radiofrequency and time-varying gradient magnetic fields.

13.2 What Physicians Working in ED, Anesthesiologists, and Surgeons Should Know

The PM is a pulse generator, generally placed in the left (less frequently right) subclavian region, usually subcutaneously or under the pectoral muscle. It is connected with the heart across the cephalic, axillary, or subclavian vein by one or two leads reaching the right ventricle, the right atrium, or both; in patients with cardiac resynchronization therapy (CRT), another lead is positioned in a branch of the coronary sinus for left ventricular pacing. Depending on the needs of an individual patient and model of the PM, programming and pacing function will differ from one device to another.

The ICDs differ from PMs for their antitachycardia properties, as they can recognize and automatically interrupt (by overdrive pacing or high-voltage DC shock) potentially fatal arrhythmias, as sustained ventricular tachycardias or ventricular fibrillation, the leading causes of sudden death. In patients with left ventricular dysfunction of any origin, as well as in those with other cardiac conditions at high risk of sudden death, treatment with ICD is associated with an improved survival even in

Table 13.1 NASPE code for pacing modalities

I	II	III	IV	V
Chamber (s) paced	Chamber (s) sensed	Response to sensing	Rate modulation	Multisite pacing
O → none A → atrium V → ventricle D → dual (A+V)	O → none A → atrium V → ventricle D → dual (A+V)	O → none T → triggered I → inhibited D → dual (A+V)	O → none R → rate modulation	O → none A → atrium V → ventricle D → dual (A+V)
S → single (A or V)	S → single (A or V)			

the absence of previous history of ventricular arrhythmias. With the exception of some newly released entirely subcutaneous ICD, without intravascular leads (s-ICD), all ICDs have PM properties. In addition, it is possible to program the minimum rate and duration of arrhythmias required to be recognized and treated, to avoid unnecessary therapies in the case of slow and/or brief self-terminating tachycardias.

13.2.1 PM Programming Modes

Pacing modalities are expressed according to the North American Society of Pacing and Electrophysiology/British Pacing and Electrophysiology Group (NASPE/BPEG) revised code (see Table 13.1) [6]. The first letter indicates the chamber in which pacing occurs, while the second indicates the chamber with sensing capabilities. The third letter indicates the effect of sensing on the triggering or inhibition of subsequent pacing stimuli. The fourth and the fifth letter, not always used in clinical practice, respectively indicate the presence (R) or absence (O) of an adaptive-rate mechanism and whether multisite pacing (as in CRT) is present.

13.2.2 Unipolar Versus Bipolar Leads

Artifacts during electrocauterization can be erroneously considered by the CIED as spontaneous fast electrical activity of the heart (oversensing) [7]. Nearly all leads implanted in the last decade are bipolar, meaning that both the cathode and the anode are on the tip of the catheter, reducing the inter-electrode distance and the likelihood of external interferences. However, in some patients, especially with less recent implantations, unipolar leads can still be present. In these patients, the risk of oversensing is particularly high, as the sensed field is included between the tip of the lead (functioning as a cathode) and the generator (anode).

13.2.3 Unipolar Versus Bipolar Electrocautery

Electrosurgery current usually occurs in the frequency range between 100 and 5000 kHz and is typically delivered in a unipolar configuration between the cauterizing instrument and ground electrode. Bipolar electrosurgery involves the use of an electrical forceps where each limb is an electrode; it is used far less commonly because it is useful only for coagulation and not dissection. Bipolar systems deliver the current between two electrodes at the tip of the instrument, reducing the likelihood for EMI with CIEDs. Therefore, malfunctions are associated with unipolar electrocautery only, while bipolar electrosurgery does not cause EMI when not directly applied to CIED.

EMI usually occur when electrosurgery is performed within 8–15 cm from the device. Electrosurgery below the umbilicus with the grounding pad placed on the thigh is therefore unlikely to result in EMI with thoracic CIEDs.

EMI are more likely with the cutting mode rather than with the coagulation mode of surgical electrocautery, probably because of the higher power and the longer period of time applied for tissue cutting than coagulating a bleeding vessel.

The use of a harmonic scalpel, an ultrasonic cutting and coagulating instrument, can avoid surgical diathermy, according to some data [8].

13.2.4 Effects of EMI on CIED: General Considerations

Depending on the type of devices and lead, the programming of the devices and the type of surgery, different malfunctions can be found.

The possible effects of EMI can be transient (due to oversensing) or permanent (initiation of noise reversion, electrical reset mode, or increase of pacing thresholds).

Permanent damages are extremely rare, unless the energy is applied directly to the pulse generator or system electrode. There are some old reports of various serious effects, such as failure to pace, system malfunction, and even inappropriate life-threatening uncontrolled pacing activity [3]. However, because of the advances in lead and generator technology, most recent reports suggest that nowadays these effects infrequently occur.

13.2.4.1 Reset
Resetting of PMs has been reported in presence of energy coursing through the pulse generator (i.e., when the electrocautery touches, or is very close to, the generator) and simulates the initial connection of the power source at the time of manufacture. During reset, pacing parameters are automatically programmed in VVI mode with a lower rate from 60 to 70/min (depending on the manufacturer) and high output energy. For ICD, beside a VVI 60–70/min pacing mode, a fixed antitachycardia therapy (with lower rate cutoff ranging from 146 to 190/min according to the manufacturer) is programmed.

13.2.4.2 Generator Damages
The application of electrosurgery either in immediate close proximity or directly to the pulse generator can cause failure or permanent damage to a CIED, especially to older pacemakers (with voltage-controlled oscillators, no longer manufactured).

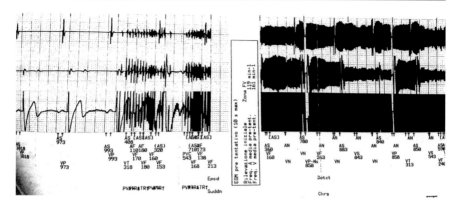

Fig. 13.1 Ventricular oversensing during thoracic surgery leading to ICD charge

ICDs may be more resistant, but energy can still enter the pulse generator in presence of breaches of lead insulation.

13.2.4.3 Lead-Tissue Interface Damage
Damage to the lead-myocardial interface is unlikely to occur with modern devices, but monopolar electrosurgery pathways crossing a pulse generator can produce enough voltage to create a unipolar current from the pulse generator case to a pacing electrode in contact with myocardium. This can result in a localized tissue damage with an increase in pacing threshold and possible loss of capture [9].

13.2.4.4 Oversensing
The most frequent CIED interaction with EMI is oversensing, leading inappropriate inhibition of pacing output and false detection of a tachyarrhythmia, with possible inappropriate CIED therapy (Fig. 13.1).

Electrosurgery applied below the umbilicus is much less likely to cause PM or ICD interference than when applied above the umbilicus. However, endoscopic gastrointestinal procedures that use electrosurgery may result in interference (Fig. 13.2). In a recent analysis on 71 subjects with ICD, EMI were recorded in 50 % of thoracic and head or neck procedures, 22 % of upper extremity procedures, 7 % of abdominal/pelvic procedures (laparoscopic cholecystectomies only), and 0 % of lower extremity procedures. No EMI in any lower abdominal procedures were recorded [10].

13.2.4.5 Pacemaker Response to EMI
When programmed in inhibited pacing modes (AAI, VVI, or DDI), pacing inhibition can occur in presence of EMI, with consequent bradycardia or asystole in PM-dependent patients. When programmed in tracking mode (DDD), sensing of EMI in the atrial channel (more likely to occur, because of the higher sensitivity necessary to detect atrial signals) could result in increased rate of ventricular pacing or false atrial arrhythmia detection and consequent "mode-switch" to inhibited pacing modes (VDI, VVI, or DDI).

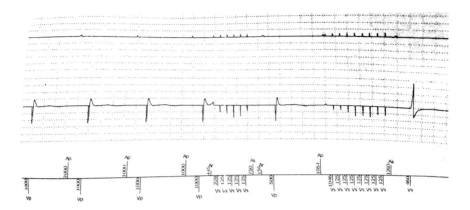

Fig. 13.2 EMI during polypectomy

For a patient with spontaneous underlying rhythm, pacing inhibition does not have any consequences, while in PM-dependent patients, a prolonged (>4–5 s) pacing inhibition can result in significant hemodynamic compromise. Therefore, *limiting electrosurgery usage to shorter bursts* is desirable and may be a safer approach than either reprogramming the CIED or placement of a magnet over the pulse generator [3].

In patients with cardiac resynchronization therapy (CRT), ventricular stimulation is, or should be, always present at surface ECG; however, these patients are not usually pacemaker dependent, so will not experience hemodynamic difficulties if biventricular pacing is transiently interrupted, with the exception of patients with advanced spontaneous AV block and those treated with AV node ablation ("ablate and pace").

13.2.4.6 ICD Response to EMI
The ICDs require a certain duration (several seconds) of continuous high-rate sensing to satisfy arrhythmia detection criteria and consequently start the treatment (antitachycardia pacing or DC shock). Therefore, short bursts (<5 s) of electrosurgery alternating with pauses lasting some seconds are unlikely to result in false tachyarrhythmia detection and inappropriate antitachycardia therapies.

Inappropriate ICD shocks, although painful in nonsedated patients, should not be necessarily considered a serious danger for both the patient (apart from skeletal muscle contraction even if the patient is paralyzed by curare) and the people surrounding, who will not experience any shock. There is, however, a rare but possible proarrhythmic effect of DC shocks, which can initiate ventricular fibrillation.

13.2.5 Effects of the Magnet

A simple magnet (typically 90 G) should always be present in the operating room when a patient with a CIED undergoes a procedure potentially causing EMI. However, the effect of the magnet positioned on the skin just above the device (Fig. 13.3) differs between pacemakers and ICDs.

Fig. 13.3 A magnet placed on the CIED pocket

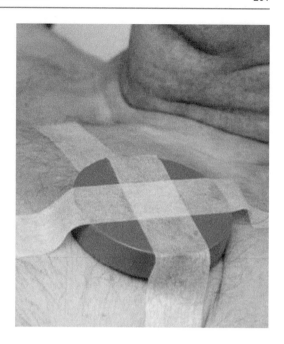

13.2.5.1 Pacemakers

When a magnet is applied on a pacemaker, it usually causes "asynchronous pacing" (generally VOO or DOO), meaning that pacing at a fixed rate is provided, independently from any sensed activity, ensuring cardiac stimulation (or avoiding inappropriate triggered activity) even in the presence of persistent artifacts. The pacing rate in the presence of a magnet is CIED characteristic and varies according to the battery charge.

If spontaneous ventricular activity is adequate, asynchronous pacing (provided by the magnet or by CIED reprogramming) can be unnecessary or even inappropriate and potentially dangerous, as the magnet rate may compete with the patient's rate; however, the risk that asynchronous pacing in patients with intrinsic rhythm can potentially induce atrial or ventricular arrhythmias, although widely feared, is very low [11].

13.2.5.2 Implantable Defibrillators

In ICDs, arrhythmias detection or tachycardia therapy can be disabled by magnet application and is automatically re-enabled when the magnetic field is removed. In some elderly Boston Scientific (former Guidant) ICDs, antitachycardia therapy may be permanently, and not transiently, deactivated by magnet application, necessitating reprogramming of the device or magnet repositioning to restore prior function. For this reason, and because it is possible to turn off magnet response in some devices, careful monitoring is required during the procedure to determine the effects of cauterization.

If inappropriate antitachycardia therapies (shock or antitachycardia pacing) should be delivered despite the magnet, shorter bursts (<5 s) with pauses between bursts, or bipolar cautery, are mandatory. On the other side, when true sustained

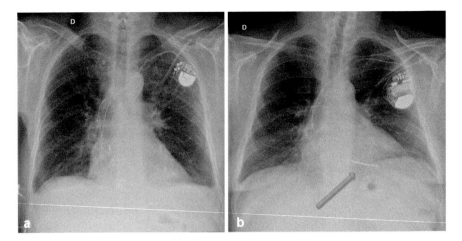

Fig. 13.4 Posterior anterior thoracic X-ray in a patient with a pacemaker (**a**) and an ICD (**b**). The shocking coil along the right ventricular lead in the ICD patient is indicated by the *arrow*

ventricular arrhythmias occur, appropriate antitachycardia therapies can be delivered by the device by just removing the magnet or by using an external defibrillator. In this case, external pads should be placed in the anteroposterior rather than anterolateral position, ensuring the anterior (apical) pad is at least 5 cm away from the device.

Differently from PM, the *magnet does not affect ICD antibradycardia pacing functions*. As a consequence, *in PM-dependent patients with ICD, reprogramming is more desirable* to avoid pacing inhibition when EMI are expected to be significant.

13.2.6 How to Recognize that a Patient Has a CIED and if Is PM Dependent

When data from medical history or files are not available, a CIED can be easily recognized by the presence of the wound in the infraclavicular region, more frequently on the left side. In less skinny patients, some devices, as some recent PMs, cannot be always detected because of the small dimensions and the position, sometimes several centimeters away from the original site under the wound.

All patients should always carry a device identification card, necessary to understand the type (PM, ICD, or CRT) and devices' manufacturer; these information are particularly important, as every device can be interrogated by the programmer from its manufacturer only. In emergency situations, chest radiograph is useful to distinguish a PM from an ICD, as the latter presents a shocking coil (section of the lead which are wider and more radiodense) along the right ventricular lead, close to the tip (Fig. 13.4). Sometimes another coil is present along the same lead, more proximally, in the superior vena cava. In addition, chest X-ray often allows the recognition of the model and even the device's serial number.

A patient with spontaneous activity is not, by definition, PM dependent. Even if the risk of bradyarrhythmias can be present, the occurrence of pauses contemporary to the inhibition of pacing during EMI is very unlikely. Therefore, PM reprogramming or magnet positioning is usually unnecessary in these patients, when the CIED is not an ICD.

When feasible, in paced patients, the PM dependence should be evaluated by the cardiologist during a preoperative PM evaluation, reprogramming the device at a low (usually 30 or 40/min) rate to detect spontaneous activity. This is particularly important in patients with CRT, where 100 % biventricular pacing is usually present, even in the absence of bradyarrhythmias. When interrogation cannot be performed before the operation, all patents with constant paced rhythm should be considered as PM dependent.

Routine PM check is usually performed every 6–12 months (3–6 for ICD). Therefore, most patients should have been evaluated in the past year; in addition, an increasing number of devices are regularly followed by "remote monitoring": using a base unit (similar to a modem), connected to the internet (via a standard phone line connection or a cell phone communication technology) and communicating wirelessly with the CIED, most information available during routing ambulatory evaluation are transmitted to designed servers and can be viewed by authorized personnel whenever desired. Data are automatically sent according to fixed intervals, in the presence of significant events (as arrhythmias or malfunctioning) or manually by the patient. Current systems, however, do not permit remote device reprogramming.

13.2.7 How to Minimize the Risk

The risk of EMI is greatest when the current field crosses the CIED or the leads or is closer than 15 cm from the CIED. During electrosurgical application, the return electrode should be placed on the ipsilateral heel or flank; however, for operations involving the ipsilateral arm of the CIED, the return electrode should be placed on the same arm to avoid the full exposure to the electrosurgical energy.

The umbilicus can be not a precise anatomical landmark especially in obese patients and many abdominal laparoscopic surgical procedures go through the umbilicus. Therefore, *iliac crest as the landmark below which no magnet or reprogramming need to be performed should be recommended. Utilization of the magnet, rather than turning off the ICDs, significantly reduces the time of exposure to the risk of untreated life-threatening arrhythmias* [10].

In addition, there is a potential risk of not re-enabling tachycardia therapies after the surgical intervention, leaving the patient unprotected in the case of ventricular arrhythmias, as demonstrated by a report on 67,410 remote follow-up patients in which the most common "red alert" was that detections and therapies for ventricular fibrillaton were "off".

Equipment for urgent cardioversion, defibrillation, and emergent pacing should be immediately available. It is important to remember, however, that artifacts can be also present at surface ECG, and arrhythmias can be difficult to detect by electrocardiographic monitoring during electrosurgical application. Therefore, cardiac activity should be monitored with other modalities, like invasive or noninvasive continuous arterial pressure monitoring or pulse oxymeter.

Therefore, *application of short burst of electrocautery (<5 s), with some seconds of pause, is the best mode to minimize the risk* of both significant bradyarryhythmias in PM-dependent patients and inappropriate antitachycardia therapy in patients with an ICD.

13.3   What the Cardiologist Should Know

When an urgent or emergent surgical intervention is needed, a cardiologist may not be immediately available, and not all cardiologists are practical with CIED programming. However, whenever possible, the cardiologist or, better, an electrophysiologist should be involved in the management of the patient, especially in case of thorax, head, or upper limbs surgery.

Clearly, the cardiologist should be aware of the patient's cardiac problems, including the reason for CIED implantation, whether the patient is PM dependent, and the model, the manufacturer, and the programming of the CIED, as responses to EMI and to magnet application vary among different CIED and according to the programming. For example, in impedance-based rate responsive systems (as in minute-ventilate sensors), EMI may result in pacing at the sensor-triggered upper rate limit if rate response is activated.

In the presence of significant EMI, a "noise reversion" may occur, during which time the CIED paces asynchronously and tachyarrhythmia therapy is suspended. Noise reversion mode is an algorithm designed to minimize the effects of EMI, and, differently from reset, it is automatically disabled once the noise is no longer present. However, noise reversion algorithms are manufacturer specific and can be useful mainly in the presence of persistent EMI; they may not provide an adequate protection in presence of sporadic and/or transient EMI, as encountered in the operating room; therefore, transient inhibition of pacing or inappropriate pacing at the programmed upper rate is more likely in this context.

13.3.1 Magnet Responses

Magnet responses vary according to different manufacturers, and different models continuously change as manufacturers release new devices. In addition, pacing rate is different at beginning of life (BOL) and at elective replace indicator (ERI).

13.3.2 Pacemakers

In PM, the magnet generally causes asynchronous pacing by closing a magnetic switch.

At BOL, VOO or DOO pacing rate vary from 85/min (Medtronic) to 100/min (Boston Scientific and S. Jude. At ERI, it decreases to lower values (Medtronic 65/min, Sorin and Biotronik 80/min, S. Jude 85–86.3/min). Other different responses can be found when magnet response is programmable (Biotronik, Boston, S. Jude).

In some devices with atrial antitachycardia therapies (Medtronic AT500), antitachycardia pacing only is suspended, but there is no conversion to an asynchronous pacing mode.

Rate response is always suspended.

In some devices (Biotronik, Boston Scientific and Medtronic), pacing amplitude remains unchanged as programmed, while if autocapture algorithm is operating, the output is usually reset above the autocapture threshold value.

13.3.3 ICD

In all ICDs, antitachy-therapy is suspended while PM functions are usually unchanged; only in Sorin devices pacing rate changes (96/min at and 80/min at ERI), continuing in demand mode (therefore, not switching in asynchronous pacing).

In some models (Boston and S. Jude), it is possible to disable magnet response to ICD.

When placing the magnet on the device, tones can be audible in some models (R wave-synchronized beep in Boston devices, steady tone in Medronic devices). However, if the device continues to emit a tone after magnet removal, it should be interrogated because of a possible fault.

13.4 A Suggested Algorithm/Pathway for Diagnosis and Treatment

13.4.1 Preoperative/Preanesthesia Assessment

In urgent/emergent setting, a preoperative assessment, as required in elective procedures, may be difficult to achieve. However, information available in the patient's records should be sufficient to generate most perioperative prescriptions, as most patients are regularly followed by ambulatory or remote evaluations.

If such evaluation has not been performed in the appropriate time frame (12 months for PM, 6 months for ICD/CRT), a consultation with an available CIED team is desirable prior to the procedure, when feasible.

13.4.2 Before Surgery

See Table 13.2

13.4.3 During Surgery

See Table 13.3

Table 13.2 Before Surgery

	What to do	How to do
All patients	Identify CIED patient	Check medical records, physical examination
	Identify the device (PM, ICD, CRT), manufacturer, and model (always)	Check medical records, patient card, or chest X-ray
	Verify CIED indications (whenever possible)	Check medical records or patient card
	Verify PM dependency (whenever possible)	Preoperatory ECG; in absence of evident spontaneous activity at surface ECG, check medical records or assume PM dependency when preoperatory interrogation and programming is not feasible
Patients with pacemaker		
PM-dependent patients *and* procedures *above* the umbilicus or iliac crest, unipolar cautery necessary	Verify underlying rhythm and spontaneous heart rate (whenever possible)	Preoperatory interrogation and transient programming at the lower rate (if not recently performed during PM routine evaluation)
	Heart rate monitoring (always)	Monitor patient with plethysmography or arterial line rather than ECG only
	Verify response to magnet placement (always)	Verify heart rate during magnet placement
	Alternative stimulation mode available (whenever possible)	Transcutaneous pacing available
Patients with ICD		
All procedures	Heart rate monitoring (always)	Monitor patient with pulse oximeter or arterial line rather than ECG only
Procedures *under* the umbilicus or iliac crest; bipolar cautery	No reprogramming required	
Procedures *above* the umbilicus or iliac crest, unipolar cautery necessary		
Magnet available and device accessible during the operation (non PM-dependent patients)	Disable antitachycardia therapies (always)	Position a magnet over the device
Magnet unavailable/device *not accessible* during the operation (but CIED personnel readily available)	Disable antitachycardia therapies (always)	Disable tachyarrhythmia therapies by programming and *ensure postoperative reprogramming*

(continued)

Table 13.2 (continued)

	What to do	How to do
PM-dependent patients (and CIED personnel readily available)	Ensure adequate heart rate	Preoperatory reprogramming in asynchronous mode (VOO or DOO) at appropriate rate and *ensure postoperative reprogramming*
PM-dependent patients; magnet unavailable/device *not accessible* during the operation; *no CIED personnel readily available*	Extreme attention to minimize EMI during electrocautery (always)	Electrosurgical return electrode placed on the ipsilateral heel or flank (or the same arm for operations involving the ipsilateral arm)

Table 13.3 During Surgery

	What to do	How to do
All procedures	Heart rate monitoring (always)	Monitor patient with pulse oxymeter or arterial line rather than ECG only
	Avoid magnetic fields (if possible)	Position sterile magnetic drapes >15 cm far from the CIED
Procedures *under* the umbilicus or iliac crest or bipolar cautery	No reprogramming required	
Procedures *above* the umbilicus or iliac crest, unipolar cautery necessary		
All patients, but particularly PM-dependent ICD patients (even with the magnet applied) ICD patients, no magnet applied PM-dependent PM patients, no magnet applied (*and* CIED personnel not readily available)	Minimize EMI during electrocautery (always)	Short electrosurgical bursts (<5 consecutive sec) with pauses >5 s
PM-dependent PM patients (magnet applied)	Verify response to magnet (always)	Verify heart rate during cauterization (with and without magnet placement)
ICD patients (therapies disabled by the magnet)	Ensure proper treatment in the case of intra-procedure ventricular arrhythmias (always)	Remove the magnet to enable tachycardia therapies
ICD patients (therapies disabled by reprogramming)		External DC shock

13.4.4 After Surgery

After surgery, CIED personnel should be contacted as soon as possible when:

- Reset of the CIED occurred during surgery.
- Reprogramming (asynchronous pacing in PM-dependent patients, disabling of antitachycardia therapy in ICD patients) before surgery was performed.
- Significant brady- or tachyarrhythmias occurred during the operation.

References

1. Wood MA, Ellenbogen KA. Cardiology patient pages: cardiac pacemakers from the patient's perspective. Circulation. 2002;105(18):2136–8.
2. Proclemer A, et al. Registro Italiano Pacemaker e Defibrillatori – Bollettino Periodico 2013. G Ital Cardiol. 2014;15(11):638–50.
3. Crossley GH, et al. The Heart Rhythm Society (HRS)/American Society of Anesthesiologists (ASA) Expert Consensus Statement on the perioperative management of patients with implantable defibrillators, pacemakers and arrhythmia monitors: facilities and patient management: executive summary this document was developed as a joint project with the American Society of Anesthesiologists (ASA), and in collaboration with the American Heart Association (AHA), and the Society of Thoracic Surgeons (STS). Heart Rhythm. 2011;8:e1–18.
4. Beinart R, Nazarian S. Effects of external electrical and magnetic fields on pacemakers and defibrillators: from engineering principles to clinical practice. Circulation. 2013;128(25):2799–809.
5. Zaphiratos V, et al. Magnetic interference of cardiac pacemakers from a surgical magnetic drape. Anesth Analg. 2013;116(3):555–9.
6. Bernstein AD, et al. The revised NASPE/BPEG generic code for antibradycardia, adaptive-rate, and multisite pacing. North American Society of Pacing and Electrophysiology/British Pacing and Electrophysiology Group. Pacing Clin Electrophysiol. 2002;25(2):260–4.
7. Dobrow RJ. Phantom pacemaker programming. Pacing Clin Electrophysiol. 1978;1:166–71.
8. Nandalan SP, Vanner RG. Use of the harmonic scalpel in a patient with a permanent pacemaker. Anaesthesia. 2004;59(6):621.
9. Snow JS, et al. Implanted devices and electromagnetic interference: case presentations and review. J Invasive Cardiol. 1995;7:25–32.
10. Gifford J, et al. Randomized controlled trial of perioperative ICD management: magnet application versus reprogramming. Pacing Clin Electrophysiol. 2014;37:1219–24.
11. Filipovic M, et al. Harm associated with reprogramming pacemakers for surgery. Anesthesiology. 2002;97:1033–4.